MANAGING THE SYMPTOMS
OF MULTIPLE SCLEROSIS

Managing the Symptoms of Multiple Sclerosis

Sixth Edition

Randall T. Schapiro, MD, FAAN

President, The Schapiro Multiple Sclerosis Advisory Group
and
Clinical Professor of Neurology (Retired),
University of Minnesota

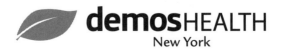

demosHEALTH
New York

Visit our website at www.demoshealth.com

ISBN: 978-1-936303-64-9
e-book ISBN: 978-1-617052-18-7

Acquisitions Editor: Julia Pastore
Compositor: diacriTech

Library of Congress Cataloging-in-Publication Data

Schapiro, Randall T.
  Managing the symptoms of multiple sclerosis / Randall T. Schapiro, MD, FAAN, President, The Schapiro Multiple Sclerosis Advisory Group and Clinical Professor of Neurology (Retired), University of Minnesota.—Sixth edition.
      pages cm
  Includes bibliographical references and index.
  ISBN 978-1-936303-64-9
  1. Multiple sclerosis—Popular works. 2. Multiple sclerosis—Palliative treatment.
I. Title.
  RC377.S255 2014
  616.8'34—dc23
                                          2014014044

Special discounts on bulk quantities of Demos Health books are available to corporations, professional associations, pharmaceutical companies, health care organizations, and other qualifying groups. For details, please contact:

Special Sales Department
Demos Medical Publishing, LLC
11 West 42nd Street, 15th Floor
New York, NY 10036
Phone: 800-532-8663 or 212-683-0072
Fax: 212-941-7842
E-mail: specialsales@demosmedical.com

Printed in the United States of America by McNaughton & Gunn.
14 15 16 17 18 / 5 4 3 2 1

To all those whose lives are altered by the effects of multiple sclerosis along with a special dedication to Diana Schneider, PhD, who founded Demos Publications and edited the previous editions of this book. She passed away after a fight with cancer but remained a major force for MS education to the end. She will be missed!

CONTENTS

Contents

PREFACE

It was not that long ago that people with multiple sclerosis (MS) were told there is nothing that can be done for them! The progress made during my career has been absolutely remarkable. When the first edition of this book was published in 1986, disease management was only dreamed about, and the backbone of managing MS was symptom management. Now, there are numerous treatments that allow for control of this seemingly uncontrollable disease for most with MS. As I have always emphasized, there is a person behind the MS who has needs that go beyond disease and symptom management, and these needs must also be addressed in any comprehensive management program.

This book remains a guide to managing the symptoms of MS, but also focuses on disease and personal management strategies. It is based on the management program developed at the oldest comprehensive MS Center in the United States, The Schapiro Center for Multiple Sclerosis (formerly The Fairview MS Center) in Minneapolis, Minnesota. With all that has happened in health care delivery, it is even more important for people with MS to take charge of their destiny as much as possible. This book provides ammunition in that fight by suggesting ways to manage the issues that accompany MS.

This new edition updates the management techniques for multiple sclerosis. A fresh look at all aspects of MS emphasizes the fact that much can be done to improve quality of life for those with the disease. It is our hope that all who use this book will be empowered to do as much as they can with what they have and to live their lives as fully as possible.

ACKNOWLEDGMENTS

I retired from practice six years ago but continue to educate nationally and internationally about MS. Without me, The Schapiro Center for Multiple Sclerosis at the Minneapolis Clinic of Neurology has continued to lead the clinical fight against MS. For almost 40 years it has seen the growth and development of organizations that have enhanced the lives of those with MS, including the National Multiple Sclerosis Society, the Consortium of Multiple Sclerosis Centers, The Multiple Sclerosis Association of America, the Multiple Sclerosis Foundation, and Can Do MS (formerly The Heuga Center).

With this new edition, the author continues to acknowledge those organizations for consistency and growth in the expansion of knowledge in MS, and especially, June Halper, MSN, ANP, FAAN (Executive Director of the Consortium of MS Centers in New Jersey), Nancy Holland, EdD (Retired Vice President National MS Society), Rosalind Kalb, PhD (the National MS Society), and Nicholas LaRocca, PhD (the National MS Society) for all they have done for those with MS.

None of this could happen without a brilliant and caring, most experienced staff of professionals during my tenure in our office: Brenda Brelje, RN, Cindy Phair, RN, MA, Rosemary Nelson, RN, Mary Grendahl, RN, and Roberta Shohn. Jonathan Calkwood, MD, continues the excellent, dedicated MS neurological care at the Schapiro Center.

The author also wishes to acknowledge the assistance of Demos Medical Publishing and its creator, Dr. Diana M. Schneider; she was an inspiration and will be missed by all. The stabilizing influence of my wife, Cathy Schapiro continues to be of utmost importance and is very much appreciated!

—Randall T. Schapiro, MD, FAAN

Part

I

THE DISEASE AND ITS MANAGEMENT

Chapter

1

WHAT IS MULTIPLE SCLEROSIS?

Multiple sclerosis (MS) is a disease of the immune system, the body's surveillance system that recognizes something that is foreign to the body and attempts to control it. In MS the immune system is very active and may see its own nervous system components as foreign and attack them. It is one of a broad category of *demyelinating* diseases that affect the *central nervous system* (CNS)—the brain and spinal cord. *Myelin* is a fatty material that insulates nerves, acting like the covering of an electrical wire and allowing nerves to transmit impulses rapidly. It is the speed and efficiency with which these impulses are conducted that permits us to perform smooth, rapid, and coordinated movements with little conscious effort. In MS the loss of myelin is accompanied by a loss of the ability to perform these movements. The sites where myelin is lost appear as hardened *sclerotic* (scarred) areas, and because there tend to be many such areas within the CNS, the term *multiple sclerosis* (literally, many scars) is appropriate.

It is well understood that the nerve fiber itself—called an "axon"—is also affected by MS. Newer studies have shown even more dramatically what has been known for hundreds of years: that the axon can degenerate in MS. This degeneration may lead to more permanent damage than if the myelin only were involved. It is also recognized that this degeneration of the axons may appear much earlier in the course of the disease than previously thought. These myelinated axons look white to the naked eye. Thus they are called white matter. It is well understood that MS is a disease of the myelin of the white matter. Now we are learning that MS is also a disease involving the other nerves, the so-called gray matter.

The brain functions somewhat as if it were a large computer or an electrical system that sends its messages down nerves in the nervous system. These nerves function like wires—you decide to move your right arm, and it moves. This amazing system is made efficient by the presence of myelin. To understand this process more completely, it is helpful to understand the anatomy of the nervous system.

A WORD ABOUT ANATOMY

The anatomy of the nerves and muscles is referred to frequently throughout this book. This overview will provide a quick reference for the reader. More specific information is included with each topic as needed.

Three fairly distinct components make up the human nervous system: the CNS, which is somewhat analogous to the main processing unit of a computer; the *peripheral nervous system* (PNS), which links the CNS to the muscles; and the *sympathetic nervous system*, which links the CNS to the internal organs (see Figure 1.1). The CNS has two major parts, the brain and spinal cord, which in turn have several subdivisions, each of which plays a unique role in regulating the functions of the body.

The portion of the brain referred to as the cerebrum acts as a master control system and is responsible for initiating all thought and movement. Memory, personality, vision, hearing, touch, and muscle tone all are housed within the *cerebrum*. Behind the cerebrum is the *cerebellum*, which coordinates movement and "smooths" muscle activity. The proper functioning of this region of

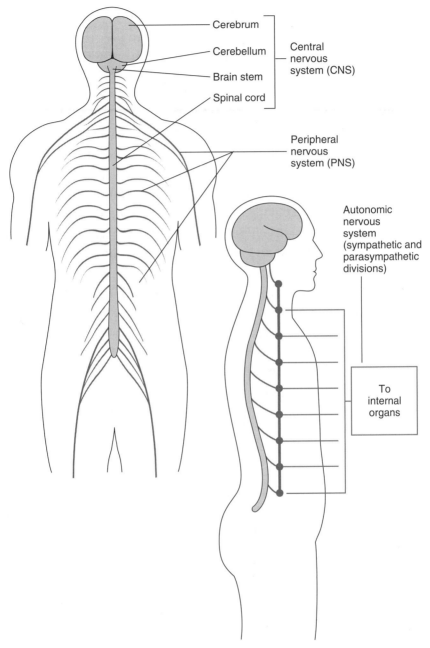

FIGURE 1.1 The nervous system.

the brain controls balance during walking and the smooth use of your hands and arms.

Beneath the cerebrum and cerebellum is the *brain stem*, which contains the nerves that control eye movements and the vital centers involved in functions such as breathing and heart rate. Extending downward from the brain stem is the *spinal cord*, which functions very much like a large electrical cord that carries messages between the brain centers and all other parts of the body. Although numerous biochemical reactions occur in the brain and spinal cord, their major role is to produce electrical activity that stimulates and regulates various bodily activities. These messages are delivered to the target structures very efficiently and effectively because the entire system is well insulated and shielded by the myelin that surrounds the conducting systems and allows the electrical nervous impulses to move through the pathways with little loss of information. The myelin in the brain and spinal cord is produced by a specific type of cell called an *oligodendrocyte* (oligo). Both oligos and myelin appear to be damaged in MS. When they are damaged, the nerve beneath the myelin sometimes is also affected (axonal damage). Oligos disappear as the affected myelin becomes hardened and scarred, forming what is called a *plaque* and causing a short-circuiting of electrical transmission.

The PNS is responsible for transmitting electrical messages between the spinal cord and the muscles, including those of the arms and legs. This system also contains myelin, although it is made by a different cell type than the oligo, a cell that does not appear to be affected by MS. Thus, although it is not uncommon to find leg or arm weakness in MS, the problem lies in the central conduction system (the brain and spinal cord), not in the peripheral nerves that lead from the spinal cord.

The *autonomic nervous system* has two divisions, the *sympathetic* and the *parasympathetic*. These systems are responsible for automatic types of function such as the beating of your heart, perspiration, and so on. This system also contains myelin, but, like the PNS, it is not directly affected by MS.

Although MS directly affects only the CNS, the disease has indirect effects on other systems and their functions because all components of the nervous system communicate with one another.

It may be stated that MS is a disease of the immune system, a disease of myelin, and a disease of axons. Most important, MS is a disease of *people*—people who have feelings that go well beyond myelin and axons. All of this leads to the reality that MS is not simple and explains why the mystery remains as to what causes this process.

SYMPTOMS OF MULTIPLE SCLEROSIS

The most common characteristics of MS include:

- Onset most commonly is between the ages of 15 and 50 years. The average age of diagnosis is 30.
- Remissions and exacerbations (improvements and flare-ups) are the rule in the initial stage of the disease.
- Scattered areas in the CNS are affected.

Because different areas of the brain and spinal cord are responsible for different kinds of movements and sensations, the neurologic deficit that results from an area of scarring depends on the exact location of the abnormality (lesion) and its relationship to other areas within the brain. For example, when an area of demyelination develops in the cerebellum, the area of the brain that is responsible for making coordinated movements, such coordination becomes difficult. Because symptoms depend on the location of the area of scarring, no two cases of MS are exactly alike, and symptoms vary considerably from one individual to another. In one person, the extent of MS symptoms might be mild disturbances of gait and vision, whereas another person might suffer a severe or complete sensory and motor loss. Some people with MS may have many, many symptoms, whereas others may have very few! In a similar fashion, some people with MS may have severe disease, whereas others may be only mildly affected.

> *No two cases of MS are exactly alike,*
> *and symptoms vary considerably from one*
> *individual to another.*

To better understand individual variations and to develop appropriate management plans, MS often is divided into subtypes. This classification also helps in having uniform groups for research studies. The most current classification includes:

- *Relapsing-remitting.* This form of MS is characterized by clearly defined acute attacks, with either full recovery or some remaining neurologic signs/symptoms and residual deficit upon recovery. The periods between relapses are characterized by a lack of disease progression. It is thought that about 80% of MS begins in this manner. Over time the course may change and then the person moves into a different category. About 50% will develop a progressive course after the relapsing start. We then call it:
- *Secondary progressive.* This form of the disease begins with an initial relapsing-remitting course, followed by progression at a variable rate that also may include occasional relapses and minor remissions. About 10% of MS worsens right from the start and is called:
- *Primary progressive.* The disease shows progression of disability from its onset, without plateaus or remissions or with occasional plateaus and temporary minor improvements. It more commonly is seen in people who develop the disease after 40 years of age. About 5% of MS starts with a progressive course and becomes more fluctuating. It is called:
- *Progressive-relapsing.* This pattern of MS shows progression from the onset but with clear acute relapses that may or may not have some recovery or remissions.

Two points should be emphasized. First, more than two-thirds of all people who have MS are walking 20 years after diagnosis. The idea that MS is a progressive disease that inevitably leads to wheelchair use does not fit the most common scenario. Second, even those who have progressive disease usually stop progressing at some point. Many MS experts fear the potential progression of the disease so much they often overlook the fact that the disease is not always progressive. About 20% of patients with MS appear to remain fairly stable. Just why this occurs is not known, despite lengthy inquiries into diet, lifestyle, and other factors. That means that about 80% of MS patients will need more aggressive management.

It is important to understand that the four classifications listed above describe the common patterns that MS takes. They are not meant to show four different diseases. Unfortunately, many insurance companies and health care plans, have adopted the idea that a person has one of these four when, in fact, people are simply put into the appropriate category by observing their patterns of disease. That may change from time to time and the person then is moved into a different category. There are other classifications used in MS that involve descriptions of the parts of the brain and spinal cord involved such as cerebral MS or spinal MS. There are also classifications based on what the disease actually looks like under the microscope. Thus the clinical classification is just one of many, and it has been overemphasized in today's world.

The MS Society has estimated that there are about 450,000 cases of MS in the United States. It is extremely difficult to estimate accurately just how many have MS because of the variability of the disease and the fact that many people can hide it or may not even recognize it. All medical professionals recognize that this data is old and should be revised in the near future. But though we truly do not know how many cases of multiple sclerosis there are in the United States or worldwide, we do know that over time we have been able to recognize it better, diagnose it easier and earlier, and understand it more clearly. This has led to earlier and more frequent diagnosis and to more certainty in the diagnosis. That gives the appearance of there being more multiple sclerosis in the world. That may, in fact, be the case, but other factors also must be taken into account.

POSSIBLE CAUSES OF MULTIPLE SCLEROSIS

Although a specific cause of MS has not yet been determined, several theories are plausible. MS generally is considered to be an autoimmune disease in which—for unknown reasons—the body's own immune system begins to attack normal body tissue. In the case of MS, the cells that make myelin, the myelin itself, and/or the axons are attacked.

The Immune System

The nervous system is not the only system in the body that "talks" to other systems and to itself. Many parts of the body communicate with each other. This is especially true for the *immune system*, which is responsible for destroying foreign substances such as viruses and bacteria. Most people know about the immune system because they are familiar with the acquired immunodeficiency syndrome (AIDS), in which a virus attacks the immune system and makes it inactive. In MS the picture is different in that the immune system appears to be *too* active. It sends out "messengers" in the form of specific types of white blood cells that attack myelin as if it were a foreign substance.

The immune system is made up of many different cells that function to protect the body. These cells are made and stored in different parts of the body and make a large number of *immunomodulating* substances. The combinations of cells and substances that may be formed are essentially unlimited, which adds to the complexity of the immune system. Some cells, called *B cells*, are made in the bone marrow. Some cells are made in other parts of the body, such as the thymus gland (over the heart) and the tonsils (in the throat); these *T cells* also communicate with and regulate each other. Cells that suppress reactions are called *T suppressor cells;* those that help reactions along are called *T helper cells*. It was thought that MS was a disease only of *T cells*. It has become known now that MS also involves the *B cells*. This new knowledge has spurred research into different areas of the immune system which appears very promising. Cells in the immune system that target foreign bodies for destruction are called *macrophages*. Each of these cells has an important individual function; together they create the *immune reaction*. These reactions usually are beneficial and often lifesaving, but sometimes the system malfunctions and produces an autoimmune problem. This is what appears to happen in MS, which is therefore often referred to as an autoimmune disease. Other autoimmune diseases include systemic lupus erythematosus (SLE) and rheumatoid arthritis. All autoimmune diseases involve a faulty regulation of the immune system that appears to be overaggressive and may need to be suppressed.

Many things influence the immune system, including exposure to foreign substances, stress, and life itself. A virus may turn the system off, whereas another challenge may turn it on.

Susceptibility to autoimmune diseases appears to be at least partly genetic, so that, although MS itself is not a hereditary disease, a hereditary factor may make an individual susceptible to its development. Approximately 10% to 20% of people with MS have MS in their extended families—a higher rate than would be expected by chance. But MS is not a hereditary disease in the sense that most people consider heredity. Clearly, people do not inherit MS, but they may inherit the *possibility* of developing the disease. The likelihood of developing MS in the absence of its presence in close family members is 1:2000 (0.2%). If a parent has MS, the probability that a daughter will develop the disease is 4:100 (4%), whereas a son's chances are 2:100 (2%). If an identical twin has MS, the likelihood of the other having it is 30%! Again, if MS were solely a hereditary disease, this figure would be 100%, but it does show that genetics plays some role in the development of the disease. Although these numbers are small, they are larger than would be expected if there were no genetic connection. Thus, it appears that one does not inherit MS, but may have a substantial chance of inheriting an immune system that may become overactive if it is stimulated in a specific way. MS is termed a *multifactorial disease*, which means that more than one factor is involved and that the factors must interact in a highly specific way to result in the disease process.

A distinct possibility exists that viruses may stimulate the immune system and lead to the development of MS in susceptible individuals. Although no virus has been consistently isolated in people with MS, many investigators believe that a virus originally is responsible for turning on the immune system and making it behave in this abnormal fashion. Because of this, much research is devoted to looking for a viral inducer of MS. Studies of populations who appear to be at high risk for MS fuel the idea of a viral origin. For example, the incidence of MS increased dramatically during World War II in the Faroe Islands off the coast of Scotland. Other islands off the Scottish coast, the Shetlands and Orkneys, had previously had a high prevalence of MS. The difference in prevalence between the two island groups appears to have involved British soldiers who moved to the Faroes during the war. This type of spread of MS follows the pattern of a viral transmission. However, no virus has been found, and the incidence of MS appears to have decreased in both island groups at this time.

The fact that viruses may cause demyelination is demonstrated by the viral origin of the demyelinating disease *tropical spastic paraparesis*. The search for a viral cause of MS continues. Rubeola, rubella, herpes, and human T-cell lymphotropic type I (HTLV-I) viruses all have been considered and eliminated. The herpes 6 virus was thought to be the culprit a few years ago, but no solid evidence for its role has emerged. This virus causes a childhood disease that is very common but temporary. Also closely studied was the common bacterium *Chlamydia*, which is common in humans, but which does not usually cause symptoms. Today the Epstein-Barr (EB) virus appears to be the culprit in many studies. This is the virus that is involved in mononucleosis. It is a very appealing hypothesis because it is more commonly seen in multiple sclerosis than expected. However, history shows a pattern, and so many once-suspected viruses are now no longer being considered. It is highly likely that if a virus is involved, it has disappeared from the body by the time the immune system has begun its reaction against myelin. The search for a viral cause continues and is further stimulated by the fact that environmental factors appear to be involved in the disease.

People who spend the first 15 years or so of life in areas at a distance from the equator have a much higher risk for developing the disease than do those who spend this part of their lives closer to the equator. After the first years, there is no correlation to where a person lives, but Caucasians appear to be at higher risk than people of other races. It may be that this tendency is emphasized by the fact that more people of the same racial type live at northern latitudes. They most commonly are genetically northern European, especially Scandinavian in origin. Today, we live in a mobile society, and differences between North and South are not as prominent as they once were. MS appears with prominence virtually everywhere. However, these types of observations suggest that vitamin D may have a role in MS. Data show that people living away from the equator with less sun per day are more likely to have decreased vitamin D levels. Other data indicate that having a lower level of vitamin D in the blood may make one more susceptible to MS. This has promoted a significant increase in studies on vitamin D. Thus far, this is theory only and, in fact, most people, no matter where they are living, have low vitamin D levels in the blood based on current standards. As our understanding of the role of vitamin D remains incomplete, this will be an area of fertile research in the next decade.

Our understanding of the impact of pregnancy has evolved over the past couple of decades. It had been observed that mothers with MS often had a more significant attack following the delivery of the baby. It was then assumed that pregnancy was bad for MS. However, we now know that women who have MS and become pregnant will actually have fewer relapses during their pregnancy. It may be that the immune system automatically turns down its intensity to keep from expelling the half-foreign body of the fetus. It may also involve female hormones of pregnancy. After the delivery there is a slight increase in the likelihood of attack from MS, but this is relatively small. Thus attitudes about pregnancy in MS have significantly changed and now it is most important to think about raising the child as opposed to conceiving her/him.

Research strategies that involve the immune system vary because it is not clear exactly where in the immune process the abnormality occurs. Thus, researchers point to many different areas of the immune system in an attempt to change what happens in the MS process.

Even if a cause of MS is not found, it may be possible to halt this disease by intervening somewhere in the immune cascade and halting its progression. This does not mean that a management strategy aimed at allowing a person with MS to do as much as possible given his or her present level of function cannot be developed. This is the principle that underlies symptom management, which has advanced with time, experience, and research. That is what this book is about—making it possible for people with MS to live creative, meaningful, and enjoyable lives.

> *People with MS usually are quite healthy and have an almost normal life span.*

MS is unique in that few diseases with the potential to cause disability appear to involve only one system in the body. Except for demyelination, oligo loss, and secondary axonal (nerve) death within the brain and spinal cord, MS leaves the individual relatively unscathed. Thus, people with MS usually are quite healthy and have an almost normal life span.

CHOOSING YOUR PHYSICIAN

A good relationship with your doctor is among the more important associations for a person with MS. However, finding a physician with whom you relate well may be not only difficult but also stressful.

Some basic principles should be understood when making a decision about the right doctor for you. Despite the fact that insurance companies and other health care plan administrators act as if one physician is the same as another, this simply is untrue. Family physicians are trained to take care of general problems, but MS is not considered a general medical problem. A person with MS does need a general physician, but clearly he or she also needs someone more specialized. Internists specialize in many complicated medical problems, but most of them probably have seen few cases of MS. Physiatrists are specialists in rehabilitation and are increasingly involved as MS doctors, especially for those who have significant disability. However, neurologists—physicians who specialize in diseases of the nervous system—usually manage MS. Today, appropriately trained clinical nurse practitioners and physician's assistants are often involved in MS care. On-the-job training has become extremely important. It matters little what we call the specialist involved. What matters more is that they have, in fact, specialized knowledge.

Not all neurologists are the same. Although neurologists are trained to make detailed and difficult diagnoses of neurologic disorders, many of them are not particularly capable of, or interested in, managing a disease after it has been diagnosed. The person with MS needs to work with a physician who will care for him or her on a long-term basis. People with MS *deserve* specialized care, but choosing a professional caregiver is not always easy.

Several factors should be considered in making your decision. Although all physicians want to be helpful, some personalities simply do not mesh. Some patients want their doctor to tell them what to do, whereas others want more choice in the process. Neither is intrinsically good or bad, but if you are with the wrong type of physician, the personal chemistry might not allow for an optimal experience. Try to be aware of the type of person you are and try to find a physician with whom you are compatible.

Remember that a patient who wants to entirely direct his or her own care is wasting money by paying a physician for advice.

A physician who takes care of himself is said to have a fool both for a patient and for a doctor. Likewise, a patient should not try to direct specialized medical care. A healthy dialogue, with the patient ultimately in control, usually works best.

Another thing to remember is that good physicians are busy. All patients would like their physician to spend a lot of time with them, and that is a fair expectation. However, just how much time is enough may be difficult to determine. Before visiting your physician, write down the specific questions that you want answered. Get right to your questions because they may raise other important questions from the physician. It helps to have a list of all your medications and their dosages, because your physician may not be aware of all the medications that you are taking.

Do not expect your doctor to fix everything that is wrong. It is hoped that he or she will be able to help with problems, but you should have realistic and attainable expectations.

There may be no physician in your area who is understanding, capable, and competent to meet your needs. If not, go outside your area to find a physician. Talk with other people who have MS and try to discover where your needs may be met. Although it is vitally important to have a relationship with a specialist, it may not be necessary to see that specialist more than once or twice a year. It is important to see your MS physician at least once a year to develop a strong and understanding relationship. It also is important to be able to contact his or her office with questions that arise between appointments. Because you know each other, a phone call often can save a visit.

Remember that medications prescribed by your physician may or may not be helpful. Do not categorically condemn all medications as unnatural and useless. Before the advent of modern medicine, the life span of many people with MS was not much beyond 40 years of age, whereas people with MS can now expect to have a reasonably normal life span. Medications should not be taken without a purpose, but they should not be feared if they are used properly.

MS is a highly variable disease, and no single management program fits everyone. It is difficult for people who are distant from problems to grasp the total picture. Insurance review organizations, businesses, and others who would like to manage care have an especially difficult time with MS. They often like to force patients to see physicians whom they know well but whom the patient may not know at all. In the case of a chronic disease such as MS, the physician–patient relationship should not be taken lightly. It may be important to attempt to get your managed care company to recognize your special problems and to make allowances for them. The squeaky wheel gets the oil, so keep squeaking until you get what you need.

A Word About Complementary Medicine

There is a lot of talk about "alternative" or "complementary" medicine as many people seek answers to the unanswerable. MS is a disease in which most people actually do well even if they do not expect to. This means that no matter what treatment one takes, a good result is likely. However, it may not be the result of the treatment, but rather of the natural history of the disease.

All of us have heard of miracle cures attributed to bee stings, lightning, cobra venom, hyperimmune cow's milk, magnets, hyperbaric oxygen, vitamins, food supplements, special shoes, calcium, and other similar "treatments." None of these have undergone research studies that support their use. All rely solely on testimonials. Gullibility does not come with MS, but it often comes with being human.

Several questions should be asked about a proposed treatment:

- Has a properly performed research study demonstrated positive results?
- Has that study been repeated in some fashion?
- Is one person or a small company making a large profit from the treatment?
- Is the treatment rational, or is it "pie in the sky"?

Even if a treatment appears ridiculous, some people will swear by it. That is human nature and will persist despite significant advances in modern medical science. There always will be people who are willing to forsake science for quackery.

Having said that, there are many treatments that are not "medical" but that may have some effect on the management of some symptoms of MS. Many of these are mentioned in later chapters and include biofeedback, meditation, relaxation, acupuncture for pain, chiropractic for back pain, and others. The appropriate use of these modalities may be helpful and should not be discouraged. We now live in an era with treatments that can change the course of MS. Using complementary supplements along with good medical approaches makes sense. Using alternative approaches that have no scientific or reasonable studies behind them instead of good medical approaches makes no sense at all. A good basic guide is *Complementary and Alternative Medicine and Multiple Sclerosis, Second Edition* by Dr. Allen C. Bowling (see Appendix D).

Chapter 2

FOR THE NEWLY DIAGNOSED

If you are newly or recently diagnosed, your head is probably swirling with information and questions. Many of these are answerable but some, unfortunately, are not. MS is not a new disease. It has been around for centuries and yet we have many unanswered questions such as: "What causes MS?" "Why me?" "How do we cure it?" and "What about what I heard from a friend that it is all about diet?" No one wants MS, just like no one wants any chronic disease. However, if there was no avoiding getting a chronic disease, MS would not be the worst one to get. Today, there are management strategies to slow the disease process, manage the symptoms, and help the person with it. It is extremely important to remember that *every single person with MS is different.* That is not just a saying but is clearly true. That means that there is no single treatment that is appropriate for everyone with MS. Professionals must keep alert to not stereotype those with MS. Much has been written in the past about "an MS personality." There is no such thing. Everyone comes with their own personality and their own reactions to the stresses of MS. Trying to find the right therapy for the right person at the right time can be challenging. It is well worth the effort to find the appropriate therapy and make it work.

When initially diagnosed, education is extremely important. Just where the education comes from makes a difference. Don't make the huge mistake of accepting information from sources that are less than reliable, including people who make up information as they go, usually to sell a product. You risk losing valuable time. There are many reliable sources available, including your health care professional. Organizations such as the National MS Society, the Multiple Sclerosis Association of America, the Multiple Sclerosis Foundation, and Can Do MS are also reliable sources of easy-to-understand information.

When initially diagnosed, you may find a support group to be helpful. They are usually available through the National MS Society in your area. Others do not relate well to this approach. Again, everyone is different. Viewing disability in others can be frightening even though you may never reach that level of disability yourself. However, being in contact with others who have MS may be beneficial and provide a deeper appreciation of the fact that each person with MS is different and yet still a person with the same need of affection and right to respect.

As you embark on management of MS, I encourage you to:

Stay active and mobile. As much as possible, continue to go to work, meetings, restaurants, movies, and church, and do all of the other activities that enrich your life, keep you connected to others, stimulate the brain, and enable the body to function better. If mobility becomes impaired, do not be afraid of assistive devices. Use whatever you need to use to stay active and keep mobile.

Be patient. Some clinicians have taken to the idea that MS should be treated as if it were cancer or HIV/AIDS. The concept is to hit it very hard up front, sometimes with multiple drugs, and stamp it out. The problem is that MS is none of those diseases and these aggressive techniques could potentially harm the individual, not only immediately but down the road. That person may well live a fairly normal life without that approach. Again, *each person with MS is different!* For some with an especially aggressive form of MS, this approach makes sense, but they are in a very small minority. MS teaches patience, as treatments rarely work immediately. It takes time to see whether the course of MS is altered by whatever treatment is being utilized. Patience is a virtue in managing MS.

Be optimistic. Recent years have brought numerous new treatments for MS, and more are on the horizon. The future of MS research is bright. Look ahead with optimism.

C h a p t e r
3

MANAGING THE DISEASE PROCESS

The management of MS has changed dramatically in the past two decades as newer agents that can actually change the course of the disease have been introduced. We recognize that we cannot predict the future with anyone, let alone those with MS, but it appears that about 20% of those with clear MS will do well with their disease no matter what we do. This figure is often debated, and much data are used as evidence for both sides of the debate, but 20% is a reasonable figure. The problem is determining who is going to be in that 20% versus the 80% who will not do as well.

Studies and now experience indicate that the medications available for altering the disease course actually make a difference. At this time, 10 FDA-approved treatments for the relapsing pattern of MS have been approved. There are two types of beta interferons: interferon beta 1b (Betaseron®, Extavia®) and interferon beta 1a (Avonex®, Rebif®). *Interferons* are proteins that the body makes in response to a foreign substance. If one gets a cold or sore throat, the body makes interferon, which then modulates the immune system. Interferons are grouped into three broad categories: alpha, beta, and gamma. Gamma interferon appears to stimulate the immune system and makes MS worse. Beta interferon appears to settle it, and it decreases the attack rate, decreases the severity of attacks, increases the time between attacks, and decreases the damage to the nervous system as monitored on magnetic resonance imaging (MRI) scanning.

Glatiramer acetate (Copaxone®) is a polypeptide—a combination of four amino acids whose structure in some way fools the immune system. It also decreases the attacks and decreases MRI damage over time.

Mitoxantrone (Novantrone®) is a chemotherapy agent, a broad suppressor of the immune system, also used to treat cancer.

Natalizumab (Tysabri®) is a once-monthly, intravenous (given into a vein) monoclonal antibody designed to hamper movement of potentially damaging immune cells from the bloodstream, across the "blood–brain barrier" into the brain and spinal cord.

Fingolimod (Gilenya®) is an oral preparation that appears to act by blocking certain receptors, found many places in the body, called sphingosine 1 phosphate receptors. By doing so, the immune cells find themselves trapped in the lymph nodes, unable to reach their targets in the central nervous system.

Teriflunomide (Aubagio®) is an oral preparation that modulates the immune system by blocking an enzyme, dihydroorotate dehydrogenase. This inhibits protein synthesis and decreases the immune system's attack on the nervous system.

Dimethyl fumarate (Tecfidera®) is an oral preparation that has an unknown mechanism of action in MS, though it is thought to inhibit immune cells and molecules. A chemically related compound has been used to treat psoriasis because of its anti-inflammatory properties.

The development of so many new medicines for the treatment of the relapsing form of MS has made it more difficult to choose which medicine is right for which person at which time. Each treatment has a tremendous amount of marketing behind it. There is a tendency to minimize the risks and only look at the benefits. It is incumbent upon all of us to keep a level head in deciding which medicine is appropriate and for whom.

These medications are expensive and have potentially serious side effects (discussed later). Care must be taken in making decisions regarding their use. There is also some controversy as to when in the course of the disease they should be introduced. Most MS experts believe that early intervention with one of these disease-modifying treatments is appropriate. The question is: How early is early? Some feel that treatment should be initiated when the diagnosis of MS is made or even suspected. They point out that a study done on those with the suspicion of MS resulted in a delay to the actual diagnosis and potentially disability. Those who have had a first attack of what appears to be consistent with MS cannot actually be diagnosed with MS until the second attack; they have been labeled as having a "clinically isolated syndrome" (CIS). Unfortunately, we do not know exactly what that means for most people with the disease, because the timing of the diagnosis may or may not have anything to do with future disability. Understanding that about 20% of people with MS may not need treatment because they will do well without it also must play a role in the decision-making process.

Much has been made of the fact that we can see abnormalities in the MRI scans and that the scans can change over the course of the person's life with the disease. Some of what has been publicized is exaggerated. Clearly the MRI is an excellent tool to be used in making an early diagnosis of MS and in helping to confirm the diagnosis. However, few hard data allow us to project the course of MS from the MRI. It is fair to assume that if there are many abnormalities on the initial scan, problems with function will be forthcoming. Beyond that, much is speculation. Clearly the scan changes over time, sometimes actually improving. What that means down the road is not known. Some feel that routine checking of MRI scans will give information about the future course of the disease, but that is not based on reality. Some feel that the brain of a person with MS will shrink if treatment is not instituted immediately. Of course, all our brains shrink with age, but it is really impossible to speculate at the front end of the diagnosis how much shrinkage will or will not occur.

Thus, many unanswered questions remain that deserve an answer and undoubtedly will be answered in the future. In the meantime, there will be some disagreement as to which agent should be given, when, and to whom. Clearly, this question must be answered by the physician who knows you and is monitoring your MS.

Treatment agents differ, even the interferons. High-dose interferon (Betaseron®, Extavia®, Rebif®) appears to be stronger than low-dose interferon (Avonex®), which is a function of dose rather than the structure of the medication, because Avonex® and Rebif® are structurally identical. No study shows that everyone with MS needs a high dose. Clearly, many people with MS can be successfully treated with a low dose, but many will need a higher dose with time. This is no different from other diseases treated with multiple medications (high blood pressure, infections, etc.).

It appears that glatiramer acetate (Copaxone®) is as effective as the interferons and, in my opinion, falls between high-dose and low-dose interferon in terms of "potency." It has fewer side effects and is well tolerated.

Natalizumab was the first of a new breed of potential treatments for MS called monoclonal antibodies. These antibodies block specific areas of the immune system, slowing the attack process seen in MS. With these specific potent approaches there is the potential of significant side effect risk. By decreasing the body's immune system significantly, the ability to fight off certain viruses decreases. One of these leads to the disease called progressive multifocal leukoencephalopathy (PML). Susceptible individuals on Natalizumab (Tysabri®) have an increased risk of developing this destructive neurological disease. While there are ways to help determine who is susceptible, this really emphasizes the concept of risk versus benefits when selecting an appropriate disease-modifying treatment (DMT). It is quite clear that the risks versus benefits of each of these DMTs must be assessed individually.

As more and more treatments for the management of multiple sclerosis become available, it will become necessary to determine the long-term risks of each. Unfortunately, at this time-many, if not most of those risks remain unknown. However, if the disease, MS, itself is worsening, the risks become worth the benefits.

Which treatment should be given and when it should be given are medical decisions that should be made by your physician with input about your lifestyle, desires, and risk comfort level. The route of administration, the frequency of dosing, the monitoring requirements, the cost of the treatment, and the insurance coverage all play a role in determining which medication might be chosen. However, the most important determining factor is how active is the disease, and what is the most appropriate treatment for that particular circumstance given the risks versus benefits.

All symptoms do not appear to have the same prognostic meaning. Numbness, tingling, dizziness, blurred vision, and pain do not seem to indicate a bad prognosis, while weakness, clumsiness, cognitive disturbance, lots of abnormality on initial MRI, and older onset (age 55 and up) may lead to more rapid progression.

The National Multiple Sclerosis Society (NMSS) has developed a practice guideline stating, in summary, that those with MS should be treated as soon as a diagnosis is made and a relapsing course (characterized by "attacks" and "remissions" with ongoing activity to the disease) is established. The Society also states that changes in medication use to fit the situation should be allowed by those paying for the treatments. None of these decisions should be casual and all need the attention of the person with MS and the medical professionals involved.

The physician's philosophy regarding disease management plays a major role in determining the treatment pathway. Because of the variability of MS, often there is no study that fits the situation exactly. Thus, many generalizations are common. There are physicians who do not treat progressive MS because they feel there is a lack of good data to guide the choice. On the other hand, if the process is clearly *progressive,* it would seem that trying reasonable approaches that have worked in other situations makes some sense. Applying the principles of immune modulation in these circumstances would be a different approach than saying nothing can be done.

Intense modulation of the immune system with high-dose beta interferon may slow the disease in the progressive phase. Immune suppression with chemotherapy agents such as mitoxantrone (Novantrone®) also appears to slow progressive MS. Novantrone® is fairly easy to administer, because it is given every three months as an intravenous injection. Occasionally some nausea, some hair loss, and some blue discoloration of the urine and the whites of the eyes occur. The major drawback appears to be that the medication accumulates in the body and—if it is necessary to treat for more than 2.5 years—the risk of the medication permanently damaging the heart increases. Thus, care must be taken. Nonetheless, if the disease is progressing to an uncomfortable degree, there is comfort in the existence of agents that can apply the brakes. As time goes by we are learning better how to apply these agents.

There are other ways to alter the immune system, and each has a scientific basis for its ability to alter the course of MS. One can remove the immune antibodies mechanically by a technique called *plasma exchange.* Unfortunately, they re-form and need to be removed at intervals. This is a very expensive management tool, but it can be utilized for refractory attacks that steroids fail to manage. One can remove the cells that attack the immune system with a process called *lymphocytapheresis.* Again, this mechanical technique has some scientific validity, but it is expensive and cumbersome and must be continually applied. Bone marrow or stem cell transplantation makes sense if one believes that the faulty immune system can be replaced and fixed. Unfortunately, more studies need to be completed to allow appropriate analysis of this dangerous, aggressive technique; death is a potential side effect of extensive immune suppression.

One cannot underestimate the power of rehabilitation as a management tool for all types of MS. This basic tenet is present in most chapters in this book.

There has been a tendency among physicians to empower their patients by letting them choose their own therapy. That has a tendency to relieve physicians of their responsibility in advising their patients as to an appropriate therapy for them. There is no question that in the end the patients must understand and agree with the therapy for it to be consistently taken. However, patients need to demand from their physicians help in the selection process, as that is what they are paying for. Simply handing out several marketing kits does not constitute that help.

THE MANAGEMENT OF SIDE EFFECTS

The use of immune-modulating medication has led to a whole new topic of discussion, that of side effect management. It should be emphasized that *none* of the immune modulators (as distinguished from immune suppressants) usually has severe side effects. The incidence of side effects forms a bell-shaped curve, showing some who have no side effects while others have many. Most have some side effects that clear over time.

Glatiramer acetate has the fewest side effects. Its daily subcutaneous injection usually causes some redness and itching at the injection site when treatment is initiated. That usually lasts about 20 minutes and often stops after a few weeks. Occasionally, increased stiffness occurs. Hives sometimes indicate an allergic reaction. One unique side effect does occasionally occur; it is very infrequent and usually does not recur, but some people may experience a sudden warm or hot sensation throughout the body along with chest tightness, shortness of breath, and a feeling of depression. This lasts about 20 minutes and will abate. If an aggressive approach with emergency medicine is applied, different problems may arise from the treatments; thus, it is recommended that you rest for 20 minutes and try not to panic if this side effect occurs.

The interferons are known for producing flu-like symptoms. Fever, nausea, and muscle aches are common when treatment is initiated. Knowing this, it is recommended that high-dose interferon (Betaseron®, Rebif®) be initiated at a quarter of the final dose each time it is taken until the side effects abate. The dose then is increased to a half-dose until stable, then three-quarters, then full dose. This is called *dose escalation*. Medication that will lower temperature is helpful (acetaminophen, ibuprofen, etc.) given four hours before injection, at the time of injection, and four hours or as necessary after injection.

Injector devices decrease side effects to some degree for all subcutaneous treatments. Small needle injections of interferon (Betaseron®, Rebif®) lead to more skin discoloration than the longer needle injection (Avonex®). These skin reactions are diminished by the injector devices. Common sense tells us that intramuscular injections are best performed by a helper. That is not true for everyone, but it holds for most people who have any problems with coordination or weakness. If pain occurs with the injection, icing before and after may help. Anesthetic creams and the judicious use of ice can be used to numb the area prior to injection if needed. Skin reactions may respond to cortisone cream. If one develops actual skin breakdown, a decision as to whether the treatment can be tolerated must be made. With interferon therapy, blood and liver tests should be monitored for a period of time because sometimes significant changes can occur. Often we accept considerable abnormality to these, but they need watching.

The body reacts to foreign medication by producing *antibodies*. Some of these may affect the potency of the treatment. Research continues as to the true meaning of antibodies and how they can be altered. It appears that only about 20% of people will develop these antibodies and that half of those will lose them. Just how often these should be measured is not clear because their relevance in the decision making is not entirely clear. What is clear is that treatments need to be changed if they are not stabilizing the disease process. This is determined by following the relapse rate, the amount of disability, and to a lesser extent the MRI scan. If there are changes in these parameters, changes in treatment should be considered. Mitoxantrone (Novantrone®) comes with heart concerns and the rare potential to cause leukemia. It can also suppress the function of the blood and liver. Care must be taken that the i's are dotted and the t's crossed; that may be best done by a physician who is used to administering such chemotherapeutic agents (e.g., an oncologist, or cancer doctor).

As previously discussed, Natalizumab is associated with the development of virus-induced progressive multifocal leukoencephalopathy in susceptible individuals. Susceptibility can be measured to some degree by measuring a specific antibody in the blood or spinal fluid. This antibody is very commonly seen in an inactive state in many normal individuals and is activated when the immune system is suppressed significantly. Duration of treatment appears to have an effect such that one is more susceptible to activation after two years of Natalizumab. The symptoms of PML are similar to worsening MS and the MRI looks significantly worse as well, thus making for some confusion when PML initiates. Treatment of PML is to restore the immune system by stopping the Natalizumab and initiating measures to restore immunity via plasma exchange or other route. The potential for this adverse reaction is not minor and should not be minimized with over 350 cases seen thus far. However, clearly, the treatment is effective for many with MS, and if the MS is worsening the risk may well be worth the benefit. This is an important concept that not only people with MS should grasp but also their clinicians. Because this treatment is administered intravenously monthly at an infusion center, side effects are watched closely. Allergic reactions are the most common issue—some may be local and others generalized. This can be a reason to stop treatment. Antibodies against the treatment may render it ineffective, and this is seen in studies as well.

Fingolimod (Gilenya®), was the first oral agent approved and has shown itself to be a potent player in the MS arena. However, this does not come without some risk and the risk–benefit profile must be viewed with each administrative decision. An unintended problem appears in some who are susceptible to the heart (cardiac) side-effects of this treatment. Observation of the heart must be well done and long enough to provide some security that an abnormal rhythm or blood pressure drop will not occur. Unfortunately, treatment is ongoing, so one has to be vigilant over time, not just at the beginning of treatment. Because of the significant immune sup pression mechanism, untoward infections must be guarded against, including progressive multifocal leukoencephalopathy.

Teriflunomide (Aubagio®) is a new oral agent that comes from a similar agent used to treat arthritis. While the long-term issues of teriflunomide are not known as yet, this similar agent brings concern regarding potential congenital problems with babies conceived while on the agent. This appears true whether the person with MS is male or female and thus the FDA gave it a pregnancy rating of X, which means it should be cleared out of the system prior to becoming pregnant. Clearing it is no small task and requires a protocol (recipe) that your physician should give to you. Other long-term issues must be watched for over time.

Dimethyl fumarate (Tecfidera®) is the newest of the agents. It is an oral treatment that is borrowed from the psoriatic treatments in Europe. There are immunological fears associated with it, but basically they are unknown as yet. There have been reported unusual viruses in psoriasis but not in MS. Because the mechanism of action is not clear, it is hard to look forward and see what the long-term implications are to using this over time. Time will eventually give us the answers as to safety and how well it works. Bowel symptoms appear to be a bothersome initial side effect and treatments vary as to whether it is nausea or diarrhea. Medications aimed at the bowel problem are often started with the treatment. Flushing is a common side effect and usually passes over time.

The Treatment of Acute Attacks

The treatment of acute attacks involves treating the inflammation (swelling) that accompanies the attack. Cortisone medication including methylprednisolone, dexamethasone, prednisone, ACTH gel (Acthar®), and others continue to be commonly used to shorten attacks. These potent anti-inflammatory drugs diminish the swelling within the brain and spinal cord that is seen as cells of the immune system invade and attack the nervous system, They do not appear to alter the long-term course of the disease. They are clearly associated with osteoporosis, cataracts, psychological changes, skin acne, weight gain, and salt and water imbalances. Thus, their effects on acute attacks must be weighed against potential problems from the treatment.

Some doctors, especially in Europe, have brought up the question: "Do relapses really matter?" They point out that with or without relapses the disease appears to have a mind of its own and will progress at a rate unrelated to relapses. From my perspective, all one has to do is ask a person with MS during a relapse whether it matters or not. Universally, if the relapse is significant the person would like to shorten it and get on with life. In the short term, relapses appear to matter a lot, and if function is impaired, an aggressive approach toward them is appropriate. It may well be true that minor relapses that do not impair would best be treated by benign neglect. These are discussions for each person to have with his or her clinician.

In unusual circumstances, plasma exchange and the use of pooled immunoglobulin (IVIG) may be recommended to manage an acute attack. Decisions as to the amount and duration of each individual treatment must be left to the clinician who is managing the problem.

$\mathcal{P}$ *a r t*
II

MANAGING THE SYMPTOMS OF MULTIPLE SCLEROSIS

Immune system–modulating medications provide the ability to truly provide disease management. They clearly are not for everyone with multiple sclerosis (MS) and must be selected and used with expert advice. The backbone to MS management has been and continues to be the management of symptoms. Everyone with MS should be aware of the many ways in which their symptoms can be managed, with the goal of improved quality of life.

The symptoms in MS may be divided into those that are caused directly by demyelination within the brain and spinal cord, and those that are not. Symptoms that are caused by the disease itself are called *primary* symptoms. If you lose myelin in the part of the brain or spinal cord that influences strength, you will develop weakness; if you lose myelin in the part that controls coordination, you will become uncoordinated; and if you lose myelin in the part that controls sensation, you will develop numbness, pain, burning, or itching. It is quite simple to understand that the number of combinations is endless. That is why no two people with MS are exactly alike.

People who have primary symptoms sometimes also suffer from problems that are only indirectly caused by the disease; these are called *secondary* symptoms. For example, some people who are weak and stiff develop decreased movement at the joints, called contractures, and immobility can lead to osteoporosis or skin breakdown.

Chronic disease may lead to changes in how one looks at life and tackles life's stresses. It may lead to depression, frustration, or vocational and marital problems. These are called *tertiary* symptoms.

Thus, to really tackle MS, the disease process should be modified whenever it is possible to do so. The symptoms of the disease should be managed to allow better function, and the person with the disease should be helped to improve his or her quality of life.

> *Symptoms of MS may be divided into those that are caused directly by demyelination within the brain and spinal cord and those that are not.*

C h a p t e r

4

FATIGUE

To those who do not have MS, it may come as a surprise that fatigue is the most disabling symptom of MS. For those who have MS, this is not at all surprising. Part of the reason that fatigue is so common and potentially disabling relates to the fact that many different kinds of fatigue are experienced by people with MS, and it is possible to have none or all of the forms at the same time.

Fatigue may result from a whole host of factors, including sleep disturbances. Bladder frequency during the night results in a poor night's sleep and fatigue the next day. Breathing problems that may be unrelated to MS may do the same. Restless legs are more common in MS and may result in not getting to the deeper stage of sleep to allow for a restful night. Medications taken for other symptoms or for other problems may have fatigue as a side effect which becomes a magnifier. Thus, it is important to be watchful for contributions from sources other than MS and to have them evaluated and treated as needed. Appropriate studies and consultations may lead to a dramatic alleviation of fatigue.

Obviously, people with MS may develop the normal fatigue that anyone else may experience. Those with MS are not fragile, and if they overdo now and then, little bad happens. We usually treat normal fatigue with the same approach in MS as in those without MS. The idea is not to push to the point of breaking, but also not to baby oneself.

A person with MS may experience a "short-circuiting" type of fatigue. This occurs when a limb has weakness as a result of demyelination. If it is fatigued, the limb exhibits increased weakness due to demyelination. This is called a *conduction block* and is well understood physiologically. The limb will recover when the arm or leg is rested, but it may be bothersome when activities require its ongoing use. Repeatedly asking the demyelinated nerve to perform when it is short-circuiting causes fatigue. The judicious use of aerobic exercise (see Chapter 21) may help build endurance, if not strength, and thus may decrease this form of fatigue. However, overexercising with weights increases both fatigue and weakness, so a careful balance must be sought. Dalfampridine (Ampyra®) is a potassium channel blocker that allows demyelinated nerves to conduct better. Though its use has only been tested for ambulatory problems, it may also be helpful for "short circuiting" neuromuscular fatigue problems.

Management strategies also include the appropriate use of exercise and rest, with the understanding that "no pain, no gain" is simply wrong. You need to rest before "short-circuiting" fatigue becomes significant.

If a person does not remain active, muscles atrophy and *deconditioning* occurs. This is another source of fatigue. Maintaining mobility is essential! It is the answer to disability. The appropriate management strategy for this type of fatigue is to exercise and maintain mobility.

Depression (see also Chapter 23) may be associated with MS and may cause significant fatigue. This may result from not eating or sleeping well, or it may be associated with a general feeling of depression. It is essential to recognize that this fatigue is related to depression. It should be managed by aggressively treating the depression with medication and counseling.

The most common fatigue seen in MS is called *lassitude*. It is sometimes referred to as "MS fatigue." Lassitude is characterized by an overwhelming sleepiness that may come on abruptly and severely at any time of day. This form of fatigue likely is biochemical in origin.

Many have speculated that the problem involves the so-called hormones of the nervous system, the cytokines. Some cytokines appear to be elevated, associated with this type of fatigue. Medications that modify brain chemistry may be helpful. Amantadine (Symmetrel®) is an example of a medication that affects the nervous system and also has antiviral effects. The antidepressants, including fluoxetine (Prozac®), paroxetine (Paxil®), and sertraline (Zoloft®), may be useful for this type of fatigue even in those who are not depressed. These medications may not be interchangeable, with one working better for one person and a different one for another. Lassitude is a bothersome form of fatigue because a person may look well and yet not be able to function. Modafinil (Provigil®) and its newer cousin, armodafinil (Nuvigil), a neurochemical with a unique mode of action, have been shown to decrease MS fatigue and have become commonly used treatments for this problem. While their mode of action is not clear, they do work by altering the brain's neurochemistry. These are becoming the most popular antifatigue drugs in MS, but because they were not designed specifically for this purpose and are thus not approved by the FDA for such, approval by insurance is hard come by. They have a potential side effect of agitation, which should be reported to your physician immediately.

Stimulant medications sometimes may be necessary. These include pemoline (Cylert®), methylphenidate (Ritalin®), and occasionally dextroamphetamine (Dexedrine®). These medications should be used with caution because they may be habit forming and may lead to agitation. A well-timed nap sometimes is most helpful in managing lassitude. The management strategy for this form of fatigue includes rest and the use of antidepressant and stimulant medications.

A major problem in managing fatigue revolves around the fact that it is difficult to measure. The "short-circuiting" fatigue can be measured by activity level measurements, for example, distance walking, and so forth. However, the most common fatigue, lassitude, is invisible and the person is often told, "You look so good!" There are paper-and-pencil tests to attempt to measure this fatigue, but they often fall short. It can be very difficult to obtain disability (either private or Social Security) because of the difficulty proving this vexing symptom.

Even though fatigue is common and potentially disabling, it should be reemphasized that people who have MS are not fragile. Although rest may be helpful, the idea that fatigue leads to increased demyelination has not been proven. The concept that MS progression occurs if a person does not rest a great deal is also without merit. You need to listen to your body, but there always are times when a little extra push is necessary, and this is not a cause for fear.

In summary, the approach to fatigue in MS involves identifying the type of fatigue and treating it specifically. Removing any contributing causes is essential. These include infections, stress, and overutilization of some medications. While medications can help, rehabilitative techniques can also be valuable.

Occupational therapists may be helpful in teaching the concept of energy conservation to those who have moderate or severe fatigue of differing varieties. Efficiency in performing activities of daily living, which include dressing, grooming, toileting, eating, and so forth, may increase the energy available for other activities.

PRINCIPLES OF ENERGY CONSERVATION

- Balance activity with rest and learn to allow time to rest when planning a day's activities. *Rest means doing nothing at all.* There is a fine line between pushing to fatigue and stopping before it sets in. Rest improves overall endurance and leaves strength for enjoyable activities.
- Plan ahead. Make a daily or weekly schedule of activities to be done, and spread heavy and light tasks throughout the day.
- Pace activity. Rest before you become exhausted. Taking time out for five- or ten-minute rest periods during an activity may be difficult at first, but it may significantly increase overall functional endurance.

- Learn "activity tolerance." See if a given activity can be broken down into a series of smaller tasks or if others can assist in its performance.
- Set priorities. Focus on items that are priorities or that must be done, and learn to let go of any guilt that may be associated with not finishing tasks as the result of fatigue.

MINIMIZING FATIGUE BY CONSERVING ENERGY

The following are some specific suggestions for common tasks and groups of tasks that most of us need to do regularly. They take advantage of the principles described previously and are designed to conserve energy expenditure.

Kitchen and Cooking Arrangements

- Store items that are used most often on shelves or in areas where they are within easy reach to minimize the need to stretch and bend.
- Keep pots and pans near the stove, and dishes and glasses near the sink or eating area.
- Keep heavy appliances such as toasters and blenders in a permanent place on countertops.
- Have various working levels in the kitchen area to accommodate different tasks, and evaluate working heights to maintain good posture and prevent fatigue. Sit whenever possible while preparing meals or washing dishes, and use a large stool with casters that roll to eliminate at least some walking. When standing for a prolonged period, ease tension in your back by keeping one foot on a step stool or an opened lower drawer.
- Use wheeled utility carts or trays to transport numerous and/or heavy items.
- Hang utensils on pegboards to provide easier accessibility.
- Have vertical partitions placed inside storage spaces to permit upright stacking of pots and pans, lids, and baking equipment.

- If storage cabinets are deep and hard to reach, use lazy Susans or sliding drawers to bring supplies and utensils within easy reach.
- Use cookware designed for oven-to-table use to eliminate the need for extra serving pieces. Use paper towels, plastic wrap, and aluminum foil to minimize cleanup.

Meal Preparation

- Have good lighting and ventilation in the cooking area.
- Gather items needed to prepare a meal, and then sit while doing the actual food preparation.
- Select foods that require minimal preparation such as dehydrated, frozen, canned, or packaged mixes.
- Use a cutting board with nails to hold items that are being cut.
- Prepare double recipes, and freeze half for later use.
- Use electrical appliances rather than manual ones whenever possible, including food processors, mixers, blenders, and can openers.
- Use a microwave oven or crockpot to cut down on cooking and cleanup time.
- Bake rather than fry whenever possible.
- Bake cookies as sheets of squares instead of using shaped cutters.
- Slide heavy items along the countertop rather than lifting them.
- Use a damp dishcloth or a sticky substance such as Dycem™ to keep a pot or bowl in place while stirring.
- Line baking pans with foil to minimize cleanup, and soak pots and pans to eliminate scrubbing.

Cleaning

- Spread tasks out over a period of time; do one main job each day rather than an entire week's cleaning at one time.
- Alternate heavy cleaning tasks with light ones, and either get help or break major heavy-duty cleaning tasks into several steps.

- Use a pail or basket to transport cleaning supplies from room to room to save on the number of trips back and forth.
- Use adaptive equipment, such as extended handles for dusters or brushes, to avoid bending.

Laundry

- Wash one or two loads as they accumulate rather than doing multiple loads less often.
- Collect clothes in one place, and transfer them to the laundry area in a wheeled cart if possible.
- If the laundry area is in a basement, plan to remain there until the laundry is done, and have a place to relax while you are waiting.
- If a clothesline is used, have it hung at shoulder height, and place the laundry basket on a chair while hanging laundry.
- Hang clothes promptly after they are dry to minimize ironing.
- Sit down while ironing.
- Buy clothes that require minimal maintenance.

Shopping for Groceries

- Plan menus before going to the store, and take a shopping list with you.
- Use the same grocery store on a regular basis, and learn where various items are located for easier shopping; using a photocopied master grocery list organized to match the store layout is a simple way to minimize time and energy.
- Use home delivery whenever possible.

Bedroom Maintenance

- Put beds on rollers if they must be moved or keep them away from walls.
- Make one side of a bed completely, then finish the other side, to minimize the amount of walking involved.

- Organize closets for easy access by making top shelves and clothing rods low enough to reach without straining.
- Use lightweight storage boxes, hanging zippered clothes bags, and plastic boxes for items that are needed daily.

Yardwork

- Alternate tasks and incorporate short rest periods to avoid fatigue.
- Keep your garden small and easy to manage.
- Use adaptive equipment, such as handles with extensions, to minimize bending.

Infant and Child Care

- Always use your leg and arm muscles rather than your back muscles when lifting an infant or child.
- Wash, change, and dress an infant at counter height.
- Kneel while washing a child in a bathtub.
- Use disposable diapers.
- Adapt the fasteners on a child's clothing for easier dressing.
- Have a child stand on a footstool while helping him or her dress or wash.

Sitting and Desk Work

- Arrange your desk and chair heights to facilitate maintaining proper posture, which reduces slumping of the shoulders and neck flexion.
- Use a chair that has good back support.
- Arrange your office so that your file cabinets, computer terminal, and other equipment are easily accessible.
- Use small lazy Susans on the desktop for pens, paper clips, tape, stapler, and so on.
- Use a phone device that allows the receiver to rest on your shoulder and frees your hands during extended conversations.

Dressing

- Lay out clothing for the next day before retiring.
- Sit while dressing whenever possible.
- When dressing, dress the weaker side first; when undressing, undress the strong side first.
- Use a long-handled shoehorn.

Bathing

- Organize shampoo, soaps, and toiletries, and keep them together by the bathtub or shower.
- Use grab bars to assist in safely getting in and out of the bathtub.
- Use a tub bench or stool while showering or bathing.
- Always avoid hot water while bathing because it increases fatigue.

Work-related organization is equally important. Obviously each job is different and customization is necessary. Occupational therapists may be able to go into the workplace and design the necessary compensatory strategies.

Chapter

5

SPASTICITY

Spasticity means *stiffness*. It is derived from the Greek word *spastikos*, meaning to tug. It begins when demyelination occurs in the nerves that regulate muscle tone. Because many of the nerves in the brain and spinal cord regulate movement and any of them may be affected by demyelination, spasticity is a common problem in MS. The stiffness often is minimal and not bothersome. In fact, a person sometimes needs the stiffness provided by spasticity to stand or pivot. At other times stiffness may become painful and may interfere with performing activities of daily living.

Spasticity tends to occur most frequently in a specific group of muscles that are responsible for maintaining upright posture. These muscles are called *antigravity* or *postural* muscles. They include the muscles of the calf (gastrocnemius), thigh (quadriceps), buttock (gluteus maximus), groin (adductor), and occasionally the back (erector spinae).

When spasticity is present, the increased stiffness in the muscles means that a great deal of energy is required to perform daily activities. Reducing spasticity produces greater freedom of movement and strength and frequently also lessens fatigue and increases coordination. The major ways in which spasticity is reduced include stretching exercises, physical therapy, and the use of medications. If spasticity does not respond to these measures and causes discomfort, a surgical procedure may be necessary.

Reducing spasticity produces greater freedom of movement and strength and frequently also lessens fatigue and increases coordination.

The first management strategy is to alleviate associated problems that magnify spasticity. Pain or discomfort anywhere in the body will magnify spasticity. These include infection, pain, skin breakdown, and any similar process that may stimulate spasticity. Table 5.1 summarizes approaches to managing spasticity.

STRETCHING

The second management strategy is to develop a specific exercise program for stiffness. An independent stretching program based on some of the principles used in physical therapy may be used at home. Appendix B describes a basic stretching program.

A thorough stretching program includes a series of exercises that are performed in certain sitting or lying positions that allow gravity to aid in stretching specific muscles. While in the sitting position, a

TABLE 5.1   Management of Spasticity

- Treat problems that increase spasticity—infection, pain, skin breakdown.
- Develop a thorough stretching program that includes both active and passive stretching.
- Use mechanical aids (orthoses) as needed.
- Use medications.
- Use surgical management for severe spasticity that does not respond to medication.

towel or long belt may be used to pull on the forefoot and ankle to stretch the calf. While lying on your stomach, you can use the towel or long belt to stretch your thigh muscles. Certain muscles may be relaxed more effectively while one is lying on the stomach or side or while lying on all fours over a beach ball, rocking rhythmically forward and backward.

The simplest and often most effective way to reduce spasticity is *passive stretching*, in which each affected joint is slowly moved into a position that stretches the spastic muscles. After each muscle reaches its stretched position, it is held there for approximately a minute to allow it to slowly relax and release the undesired tension. Begin by lying on your back and flexing one foot to stretch the muscles in your ankle and calf. Hold the stretch for about a minute, then slowly release. Then proceed upward to the muscles in the back of the thigh, the buttocks, the groin, and, after turning from the back to the stomach, the muscles on the front of the thigh. These stretching exercises differ from *range-of-motion* exercises, which do not require you to hold the stretch for a specific length of time. Although range of motion is important, holding the stretch is significant, and patience is essential when doing the stretches.

Exercising in a pool also may be extremely beneficial because the buoyancy of the water allows movements to be performed with less energy expenditure and more efficient use of many muscles. We recommend using the pool for both stretching and range-of-movement exercises. The pool temperature should be about 85 degrees; this may feel cold to some people, but warmer temperatures should be avoided because they produce fatigue. Temperatures colder than 85 degrees can actually cause spasticity, thus the temperature of the pool is quite important.

Many people with MS have a limited range of movement in at least some joints and muscles, and the key to managing spasticity is to expand the number and kind of movements that can be performed. The exercises should be performed with a minimum of effort.

The key to managing spasticity is to expand the number and kind of movements that can be performed.

Spasticity also may be reduced by relaxation techniques that involve a combination of progressive tensing and relaxing of individual muscles, accompanied by deep breathing techniques and imagery. Acupuncture may also decrease spasticity for some people, although the mechanism of action of this is not known.

MECHANICAL AIDS

Specific devices sometimes are made for certain individuals to counteract spasticity and prevent what are termed contractures, in which the range of movement possible for a given joint becomes restricted as the result of spasticity. For example, a "toe spreader" or "finger spreader" is used to relax tightness in the feet and hands and to aid in mobility. Braces for the wrist, foot, and hand are used to maintain a natural position and to prevent limitations on movement and the development of deformities. These devices are called *orthoses*. An orthosis for the foot is an ankle-foot orthosis, or AFO. AFOs are made to place the foot at many different angles to the ankle. A good orthotist can make a brace to take stress off the knee. Hinges may increase flexibility. All orthoses should be customized to allow for maximal benefit.

MEDICATIONS

Spasticity often is managed most effectively by medications (see Table 5.2). Baclofen acts on the nerves that control the spastic muscles at their site of origin in the spinal cord. It is the most common antispasticity medication used in MS, and most people respond well

TABLE 5.2 Medications for the Management of Spasticity

Medication	Notes
Baclofen	May produce weakness at higher dose
Tizanidine (Zanaflex®)	Often combined with baclofen; may produce drowsiness
Sodium dantrolene (Dantrium®)	May produce weakness
Diazepam (Valium®)	Highly sedating; most often used at night; may become addictive
Clonazepam (Klonopin®)	Sedating; most often used at night
Cyproheptadine HCL (Periactin®)	Sedating; used primarily as an "add-on" medication
Cyclobenzaprine HCL (Flexeril®)	Used for back spasms; most often combined with other medications
Gabapentin (Neurontin®)	May ease spasms that are difficult to manage
L-Dopa (Sinemet®)	Especially useful for nighttime spasms
Ropinirole (Requip®) Pramipexole dihydrochloride (Mirapex®)	Especially useful for nighttime spasms
Carbamazepine (Tegretol®)	Used for flexor spasms of the arm or leg
Cortisone	Effective for paroxysmal spasms; should only be used on a short-term basis

to it. The dose must be carefully determined for each individual; too little will be ineffective, whereas too much produces fatigue and a feeling of weakness because it interferes with the proper degree of stiffness needed for balance and erect posture. The correct dose usually is determined by starting at a low level and slowly increasing the dose until a maximal beneficial effect is obtained. The most common mistake when taking baclofen is to give up on it too soon, so that the dose never reaches the level necessary to attain proper relaxation. That dose may be as low as one-half of a pill (5 mg) per day, but some people may need to take as much as 40 mg four times a day. Baclofen is only available as a generic and may be the least expensive medical treatment for spasticity, so it is often the initial drug used. The metabolism of baclofen in the body is relatively quick, and frequent dosing is usually necessary. This is best done by allowing each person to understand how the medication affects his or her body and tailoring it individually.

Tizanidine (Zanaflex®) acts on a different area of the spinal cord than baclofen. It appears to be effective in decreasing stiffness and muscle spasm, with less effect on strength than many other drugs. It must be used carefully and slowly because sleepiness inevitably results if the dose is increased too rapidly. The starting dose is 2 to 4 mg up to a maximum of 36 mg per day. It is quite effective and may be combined with baclofen in problem situations. It is especially useful for nighttime stiffness and spasms.

It is not uncommon for the night to be the worst time for stiffness and spasms. This appears to have something to do with the lack of outside stimulation to the nervous system, making it more sensitive to spasm. This nighttime exaggeration of muscle tone may manifest itself as restless legs. Medications that decrease restless legs may be very useful during the night. These include the medications used in Parkinson's disease, including pramipexole dihydrochloride (Mirapex®) and ropinirole HCl (Requip®). L-Dopa (Sinemet®) is another Parkinson's medication that also decreases spasms, especially the painful spasms that tend to occur at night and may become especially prominent and painful.

Diazepam (Valium®) also relieves spasms that occur at night. Its calming effect also helps to induce sleep, but its strong sedative effect limits its use during the daytime. Diazepam must be prescribed with caution because it may become addictive if used too frequently. Clonazepam (Klonopin®) is closely related to diazepam. Its main use has been to treat certain types of epilepsy. It produces significant relaxation, and thus may be used as an antispasticity medication. Like diazepam, it sedates and is best used at bedtime. When using diazepam or clonazepam, both the doctor and the person with MS must pay attention to the potential for chemical dependency. When properly used at appropriate doses, this is not a major problem. However, if the dose must be continually increased and the person is using the medication not for spasticity but as a crutch to escape the realities of the world, it should no longer be used.

Another medication that sometimes is used for spasticity is sodium dantrolene (Dantrium®), which acts directly on muscles. It is a very potent medication that needs to be used carefully. it may be helpful, but it also may induce weakness, even at low doses.

Cyproheptadine (Periactin®) is an antihistamine that has antispasticity properties and may be a good add-on medication at certain times. Its sedating effect limits its use, but doses of 4 mg taken when needed may be helpful.

A drug that is commonly used for spasms in the muscles of the back is cyclobenzaprine Hcl (Flexeril®). It acts quite specifically on these spasms, but also may relieve limb spasms. It usually works best in combination with one of the other antispasticity medications.

Gabapentin (Neurontin®), lamotrigine (Lamictal®), topiramate (Topamax®), and pregabalin (Lyrica®) are examples of newer medications that have been approved for use in seizures. These medications also have antispasticity properties, and when taken in appropriate doses often ease problematic spasms.

Any of these medications may become less effective when they are taken for a prolonged period (this is referred to as the development of tolerance), and it may be necessary to stop taking them for a period of time, after which they may again become effective.

Marijuana has not been approved by the FDA for use in MS. Nonetheless several states have approved the use of "medical" marijuana. Studies have shown some effect on spasticity with the inhalation of cannabis. These studies are not of the quality that would allow FDA approval and lack the concern about the potential damage to the lungs seen with inhalation of marijuana that make its general use impractical. There is a medication (Sativex) that is in the form of a spray containing cannabis that is available in some countries but has not gotten approval in the United States as yet.

The use of marijuana in MS today rests with individuals, the laws, and their health care providers. It would seem important to actually understand the risk–benefit ratio of its use in the future.

PAROXYSMAL (TONIC) SPASMS

People with MS very occasionally develop *paroxysmal* or tonic spasms, in which an entire arm or leg may draw up or out in a stiff, clenched, or extended position. If such spasms involve both legs, they are termed *extensor* or *flexor* spasms. These spasms may be so strong that they literally propel a person out of his or her chair. Obviously this is disconcerting, but it also is potentially dangerous. Carbamazepine (Tegretol®), another drug used for seizures, generally is used to control such spasms, although baclofen and tizanidine (Zanaflex®) also may be effective. In the past few years the newer antiseizure medications available are quite effective in managing paroxysmal spasms. They include, in addition to those above, Trileptal® and Carbatrol®. Cortisone may decrease spasticity in general and is quite effective for paroxysmal spasms when it is used on a short-term basis. Its long-term use is not advocated because of numerous associated risks. The management strategy with medication is to use what works at the proper dose. Overdosing may cause increased weakness, somnolence, and decreased function.

SURGICAL MANAGEMENT

For those who have severe *intractable* spasticity, the kind that causes problems with all functions and is not responsive to exercise or medication, a spasticity-decreasing procedure may be necessary. Nerves that control specific muscles of the leg may be destroyed with *phenol*, a chemical that is injected into the muscle. This is called a *motor point block*. It is used only for the most severe spasms that do not respond to drug therapy. It may produce flaccidity in the muscles, a profound looseness that is the opposite of spasticity. This relaxation may be more comfortable, but it usually does not increase functional mobility. It becomes progressively more difficult to repeat this procedure because of technical problems.

A better, more modern technique is the use of *botulinum toxin* (Botox®, Myobloc™), made by bacteria. This paralytic agent causes a temporary blockage of the nerve and muscle. It is easier to control than phenol, but it may require more frequent injections into the muscle. It is practical for treating small muscle spasms, especially those about the eye or face, or single muscle spasms in the extremities; severe large muscle spasms may require too high a dose to be safe. Specialists have learned over time that botulinum toxin may be repetitively given in three-month intervals with significant success in alleviating very difficult spasticity. The clinician finds the point where the nerve and the muscle intersect. That is typically done electrically and the small amount of toxin is then injected into that region. Over the next day or two, the improvement in stiffness typically continues.

Severe spasms also may be managed by a surgical procedure that involves cutting nerves or tendons to decrease the contraction of specific muscles that are producing stiffness.

A better approach to the management of severe spasticity involves the use of a pump (Synchromed®) that delivers baclofen directly into the spinal canal. A tube is placed in the canal and then is connected (beneath the skin) to a pump implanted in the abdominal region. The pump contains baclofen, which is delivered into the spinal canal at prescribed levels. The pump may be programmed by computer via radio waves so that the dose may be changed as needed. For some patients this technique may provide relief for intractable spasticity. Because the baclofen is delivered directly into the spinal canal and the level in blood and tissues remains low, side effects also are very low, and there almost always is a significant decrease in fatigue and malaise. This treatment is aggressive and expensive and should be reserved for those with severe spasticity that cannot be adequately managed by oral medications. While aggressive, it has stood the test of time and experienced clinicians can select the correct person who will benefit from this treatment.

CONTRACTURES

A *contracture* is a freezing of a joint so that it cannot bend through its full range of motion. This occurs when a joint has not been kept mobile, usually as the result of spasticity. A joint that develops a contracture becomes useless and often is painful.

All of the approaches used to treat spasticity play a role in the management of contractures. The joint must be slowly mobilized, sometimes with heat or ice applied just before stretching to ease pain and allow for more efficient stretching. Special equipment such as a tilt board may be helpful. Baclofen (taken either orally or via the pump), tizanidine, clonazepam, diazepam, or dantrolene may be used to decrease muscle tone and permit faster relief from the contracture. Occasionally, cortisone is injected directly into the joint to decrease inflammation and increase mobility. Braces may be designed to slowly stretch the joint; by changing the angle of the brace over time, a frozen joint sometimes may become mobile. Serially casting the joint (as if it were broken) by slowly stretching it with the casts may be helpful. In extreme conditions surgery may be required to release the muscle tendons to allow the joint to move.

Joints usually freeze into a contracted position, but they occasionally become fixed in the extended or straight position. Although this usually is less of a problem in terms of overall function, it is not considered an acceptable outcome, and this type of frozen joint generally is treated in a similarly aggressive manner as a contracted joint.

Chapter

6

WEAKNESS

Striving for increased mobility means working with whatever strengths and weaknesses you have. Muscle weakness that results from loss of strength in a muscle or group of muscles may occur for many reasons and is common to many diseases. Weakness in the muscle itself is seen in muscular dystrophy; in diabetic neuropathy the problem lies in the nerve that leads to the muscle; and in MS it is caused by a problem in the transmission of electrical impulses to the muscle from within the brain and spinal cord. This difficulty is the result of demyelination of the involved nerves, usually in the spinal cord but occasionally in the brain.

It is vital that the source of the weakness be understood to properly manage it. For example, if weakness is the result of a lazy, weak muscle, the muscle may be strengthened by lifting weights. These exercises are called *progressive resistive exercises*. However, when weakness is the result of poor transmission of electrical impulses, lifting weights may only fatigue the nerve and further increase muscle weakness. For people with MS, it is important to realize that exercises that involve lifting weights or repetitive movements of muscles to the point of fatigue may not increase strength but increase weakness. It is somewhat akin to a light fixture that does not work because there is a problem with the fuse. Changing the bulb or flicking the switch will not fix the problem. In MS the problem is with the fuse, and attempting to correct the problem at the muscle or nerve level will only result in frustration.

> *Exercises that involve lifting weights or repetitive movements of muscles to the point of fatigue do not increase strength, they increase weakness.*

A weak muscle that is not stimulated at all will become weaker. Such *disuse weakness* or *atrophy* may happen to anyone who has had an arm or leg placed in a cast for any length of time; when the cast is removed, your muscles have shrunk. All muscles need exercise to remain functional. It is important to determine what exercises are appropriate for your specific situation. This likely will require the assistance of a trained physical therapist who has knowledge of both the neuromuscular system and the specific problems involved in MS. The problems experienced by the person with MS must not be treated as they would be if they were the result of a broken bone rather than a misfiring central nervous system. If there is sufficient nerve supply in the brain and spinal cord to allow increasing strength and muscle bulk, success with progressive resistive exercises may be similar to a normal situation. In the past several years more has been learned about increasing strength through exercise. The principles remain the same with a goal toward expanding muscle function through weight training without increasing fatigue which produces weakness. Now more than ever, a physical therapist who understands these principles is required for success.

It is impossible to separate the management of weakness from that of spasticity and fatigue. If muscles are less stiff, less energy is expended for movement. Frequently, therefore, drugs or other treatments that lessen spasticity also increase strength. However, their overuse or use at too high a dose may increase weakness. Similarly, lessening fatigue also may increase strength.

Efficiency is the key to increasing strength in people with MS. Energy should be conserved and used wisely. This means using your muscles for practical, enjoyable activities and planning the use of time accordingly. For example, difficult activities should be done before those that are easier to perform. The appropriate use of assistive devices also may be extremely helpful in increasing overall efficiency.

As noted, an intelligent approach to strengthening exercises is necessary. Strength also may be increased with the use of an aerobic exercise machine such as an exercycle or a rowing machine. However, the principle of not becoming fatigued and exercising those muscles that can be strengthened to compensate for the weaker muscles must be applied. In general, exercise is good, but the wrong exercises may be harmful.

Placing electrodes on the muscles externally and using a computer to functionally stimulate the muscles allows muscle contraction, which can build bulk. This is called "functional electrical stimulation" (FES). This concept is not new, but newer techniques are interesting. The electricity may be felt and may be uncomfortable, but as of yet this modality is not very practical in the treatment of MS.

C h a p t e r
7

Tremor and Balance

Another symptom that impairs mobility is tremor, which refers to an oscillating movement of the extremities or occasionally the head. This symptom of MS often is associated with difficulty in balance and coordination. As is true of all symptoms of MS, tremor may come and go. It is one of the most frustrating symptoms to treat. There are many different kinds of tremors; some have wide oscillations (a gross tremor), while others are barely perceptible (a fine tremor); some occur at rest, whereas others occur only with purposeful movement; some are fast, others are slow; some involve the limbs, while others affect the head, trunk, or speech; some are disabling, but others are merely a nuisance; and some are treatable, while some are not. As with all symptoms, proper diagnosis is essential before correct management decisions can be made (Table 7.1).

Balance

Balance is necessary to perform coordinated movements, whether one is standing, sitting, or lying down. It involves the function of many neurologic centers. The *cerebellum* is the main center for balance, but the eyes, ears, and nerves to the arms and legs also contribute to balance (Figure 7.1). An impairment in any of these areas may cause balance to worsen, and it may help to compensate

TABLE 7.1   The Management of Tremor

- Exercises for balance and coordination
  - patterning
  - vestibular stimulation
  - Swiss ball
  - computerized balance stimulation
- Medications
- Mechanical approaches
  - immobilization
  - weighting
  - stabilization with braces

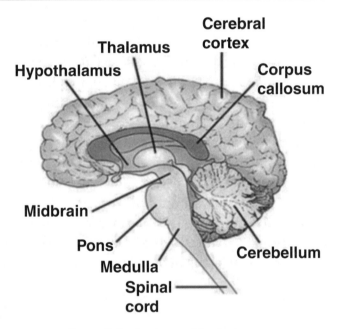

FIGURE 7.1   Anatomy of the brain.

for others that are not working properly. For example, a person with a balance problem caused by poor sensation in the feet may use her eyes to see the ground and avoid falling; obviously, this is a problem in the dark.

No medication is available to improve balance, so it is necessary to rely on exercises. Although there are no specific exercises for tremor, there *are* exercises for balance and coordination. *Patterning* refers to a technique that is used by physical and occupational therapists to trace and repeat basic movement patterns. It is based on the theory that certain muscles may be trained to move in a coordinated fashion by repeatedly using the nervous circuit that is involved in a movement. These normal movements are guided and assisted by the therapist until they become automatic. Minor resistance is then added and removed while the patient repeats the pattern independently. The muscles gradually appear to develop increased endurance for these learned movements and manage to retain control when the patterns are applied to functional tasks.

Vestibular stimulation refers to increasing the amount of stimulation received by the balance centers in the brain stem, allowing the brain to function more normally. The techniques used challenge your sense of balance by rocking, swinging, or spinning using such activities as sitting on a beach ball or swinging in a hammock. Along the same lines are exercises that are performed with a Swiss ball. This large ball may become part of a balance program designed to stimulate many different balance centers within the body.

If a person is able to stand, computerized balance stimulation with a machine dubbed a "balance master" may be helpful. The person stands on a platform that is in contact with a video screen via a computer. Movements of the feet influence the screen much like a video game, and this may be used to teach the person how to achieve better control of balance.

A number of medications may help to decrease tremor. The most common tremor seen in MS, and the most difficult to treat, occurs as a result of demyelination in the cerebellum. This area of the brain is responsible for balance and has connections throughout the brain stem (the back of the brain) and the spinal cord. Demyelination in this area often results in a gross tremor that is relatively slow and occurs during purposeful movements of the arm or leg.

This type of tremor almost always is exacerbated at times of stress and anxiety. The reason for this is not known, but exacerbation by stress is true of most of the neurologic symptoms of MS. Therefore, one mode of managing the problem is treatment with drugs that have a calming or sedative effect. For example, hydroxyzine (Atarax®, Vistaril®) is an antihistamine whose effect is to settle a minor tremor that has been magnified by stress (Table 7.2). Clonazepam (Klonopin®) also may decrease a tremor via its sedative effect. The antitremor effect must be balanced against the generally unwanted effects of sedation by carefully monitoring the dose until the desired effect is achieved.

Propranolol (Inderal®), a *beta-blocking* agent (so called because it blocks specific nerves, termed *beta fibers,* within the nervous system) is helpful in controlling certain inherited tremors, tremors of aging, and some tremors seen in MS. It is started at a low dose and increased over time until an effect is obtained. The effect may not be great, but even a small decrease in tremor may allow for greater function. Some people develop low blood pressure when they are receiving beta blockers, but this is surprisingly uncommon in the MS population being treated for tremor.

TABLE 7.2   Medications for the Management of Tremor

Medication	Notes
Hydroxyzine (Atarax®, Vistaril®)	May settle a minor tremor that has been worsened by stress
Clonazepam (Klonopin®)	May decrease tremor through sedative effect
Propranolol (Inderal®)	May provide modest relief
Buspirone (Buspar®)	An antianxiety agent that has some antitremor effect
Ondansetron (Zofran®)	May significantly decrease tremor with few side effects; cost is prohibitive
Primidone (Mysoline®)	An antiepileptic drug that may help tremor in low doses; highly sedating
Acetazolamide (Diamox®)	A diuretic that may help some people; may alleviate tremors influenced by posture

Buspirone (Buspar®) is primarily a nonsedating, nonhabit-forming antianxiety drug. For some reason it appears to have antitremor properties in MS at a dose of 5 to 10 mg, three to four times per day. It is well tolerated and may be helpful.

Ondansetron (Zofran®) may be effective for tremor, but it is very expensive. Its primary use is for the nausea that is associated with cancer chemotherapy. In a dose of 4 to 8 mg three to four times per day, it may significantly decrease tremor with few side effects.

Some studies have shown that the antiepileptic drug primidone (Mysoline®) may help manage this difficult symptom. Although it is highly sedating, low doses may be worthwhile. Acetazolamide (Diamox®) is a diuretic ("water pill") that has some antitremor properties and may be of value for some people.

Some medications, such as phenothiazine tranquilizers, may cause a tremor to worsen, and on occasion they may produce a *resting tremor* (a tremor that occurs only when a limb is not involved in purposeful movement) where none previously existed. Although their sedative effect may be useful in the treatment of a tremor that occurs with purposeful movement, the presence of a resting tremor must be balanced against the positive therapeutic effects of the drug.

Because a component of spasm often is involved in gross tremors, baclofen may provide some relief. The potential but reversible side effect of weakness must be balanced against the tremor-reducing effect of the drug, again by careful adjustment of the dose. In a similar way of thinking, botulinum toxin may judiciously be injected into the dominant muscle to decrease the amplitude of the tremor. Care must be taken to not weaken too much but to try to equilibrate.

High doses of isoniazid (INH), a medication primarily used for the treatment of tuberculosis, may alleviate gross tremors that are influenced by posture. It sometimes is worth a trial if tremor is especially incapacitating, but high doses may be too toxic in a given individual to be used for this purpose.

Occasionally, a tremor seen in people who have MS is of a type called *physiologic,* also referred to as an *essential* or *familial* tremor.

This is unrelated to MS itself and is treatable with propranolol (Inderal®).

Tremors sometimes may be helped by mechanical means. *Immobilization* refers to the placement of a rigid brace across a joint, fixing it in one position and alleviating the severity of a tremor by reducing random movement in the joint. Bracing is most helpful in the ankle and foot, providing a stable base for standing and walking. It also may be used for the arm and hand. The desired position of function is defined by the tasks that are to be facilitated, such as writing, eating, or knitting. The brace is used to immobilize the arm or hand for these tasks and then is removed.

Weighting involves the addition of weight to a part of the body to provide increased control over its movements. The general theory behind this approach is that more muscles will be used to stabilize a distant point in the body (hands, wrists, feet, ankles) when a heavier object is involved. This stabilizing action also tends to reduce tremor and to provide greater sensory feedback to the brain. In practical terms, either the limb itself may be weighted or the object being used may be made heavier, including utensils, pens or pencils, canes, walkers, and so forth.

These techniques are all used primarily for tremors that affect the limbs. The goal is to teach the person with MS to compensate for tremor by providing as much stability for the limbs as possible. It may be important to develop postural adjustments, such as setting one's arms close to the body. Adaptive equipment and/or assistive devices that are nonskid, easy to grasp, and stable are helpful and may be used for such activities as eating, writing, dressing, cooking, and homemaking.

Tremors of the head, neck, and upper torso are more difficult to manage than those of the limbs. Stabilizing the neck with a brace may be helpful.

Tremors of the lips, tongue, or jaw may affect speech by interfering either with breath control for phrasing and loudness or with the ability to vocalize and pronounce sounds. Speech therapy focuses on increasing the ability to communicate efficiently. It may involve changing the rate of speaking or the phrasing of sentences. Suggestions may be made as to the placement of the lips, tongue, or jaw for the best possible sound production. A simple paceboard, consisting of a pattern of rectangles set next to each other, may slow the person's speech and allow for improved intelligibility. The person points to each square while uttering a single syllable. A diametric increase in clarity of speech often results if he or she can slow down to keep pace with the pointing. A paceboard may be very simple, effective, and inexpensive. In some cases, tremor may make it impossible to speak, in which case alternative communication devices must be used.

None of these techniques completely eliminates the problems of tremor. The goal is continued function, which often may be accomplished by combining some of these therapies.

Surgery for tremor has become relatively popular in Parkinson's disease. Placing a stimulator or making a small lesion (scar) in the brain may decrease the Parkinson's tremor, and it is thought that it could be helpful in MS as well. There have been several reports of success in utilizing this technique in MS. The major issue is that the procedure itself and the electrode placed may increase demyelination. For severe tremor this may be the last resort. Surgeons who do this type of surgery must be aware of the issues in MS that differentiate it from Parkinson's. This may be very successful for a highly selected population of patients.

Chapter

8

PAROXYSMAL SYMPTOMS

Paroxysmal symptoms come repetitively in waves involving muscle contractions or unusual sensations. They occur relatively uniquely in MS and can be confused with seizures such as those seen in epilepsy, but are not associated with a short-circuiting of brain waves as is epilepsy. Most commonly seen is a spasm of an arm or leg that recurs every few seconds or minutes and lasts for seconds each time. Sometimes the spasm affects the muscles used to produce speech and there is a "paroxysm" of slurring. This can also occur with swallowing. Occasionally, numbness or pain occurs in a wave (see also Chapter 16), called a "neuralgia." The pain is lancinating and severe, and when it occurs in the face it is called "trigeminal neuralgia." Sometimes surgery is necessary to calm the firing nerve. This surgery may leave numbness in the area but does not disfigure the face with weakness. Sometimes the pain can be in other parts of the body, but what is consistent is the coming-and-going nature of it.

These symptoms can be frightening and often are misdiagnosed as something else. What is important to recognize is that they are usually fairly easily treated, but do require the use of appropriate medication. The older antiepilepsy drugs phenytoin (Dilantin®), valproate (Depakote®), and carbamazepine (Tegretol®) still are useful, but now many more medications are available, including gabapentin (Neurontin®), pregabalin (Lyrica®), tiagabine (Gabitril®), levetiracetam (Keppra®), and oxcarbazepine (Trileptal®). There are also improved versions of older treatments, including Carbatrol® for carbamazepine and Depakote ER® for Depakote®. A short treatment with steroids may aid in controlling the problem.

The appropriate dose for each drug varies with the individual, and an experienced clinician should manage each treatment to ensure appropriate use of the agents. While the symptoms can be frightening, they are usually self-limiting and will go away on their own with time; these symptoms are not likely to require a lifetime of treatment. The drugs should be reduced gradually after the symptoms are controlled to see if they still are necessary. If the symptoms recur, the treatment should be continued.

9

MOBILITY: PUTTING IT ALL TOGETHER

Mobility is the key to living optimally despite a disability. To function in society today one must remain mobile. To remain mobile it is essential to get the right equipment and learn how to use it. It must be stressed that using the various devices available gives you the opportunity to remain mobile. The tools to help you stay mobile have dramatically improved in the past decade. Today's walkers are

> *The answer to disability is mobility!*
> *To remain mobile it is essential to get the*
> *right equipment and learn how to use it.*

not "your mother's walker." Today's power chairs are marvelous and allow for a new world to be opened to you. Your attitude toward the use of mobility devices needs to focus on the multitude of advantages they offer.

WALKING (AMBULATION)

Movement impairment frequently is associated with MS, and difficulty in walking is a major type of such impairment. Walking is an activity that we value, perhaps far beyond its true value. Walking usually is done to get somewhere—it is a means of transportation. If walking becomes impaired, another more practical means to accomplish the same goal should be substituted, ideally without too much emotional trauma. This is easy to say but more difficult in practice. However, understanding *why* we walk may help when selecting appropriate devices to aid in walking.

Weak foot muscles may cause *a foot drop,* in which the toes of the weak foot touch the ground before the heel, thereby disrupting balance. Because there is no way to strengthen a weakened foot, compensation techniques become essential.

It is particularly important to wear proper shoes. I recommend a leather-soled oxford. The laces give maximum stability to the foot, and the smooth leather sole prevents the sticking that often occurs with crepe or similar types of soles that can throw you off balance. Leather soles wear with time and need to be replaced rather frequently, but their advantages far outweigh this minor problem. A plastic (polypropylene) insert often is added to the shoe to keep the foot from dropping. This lightweight brace (an ankle-foot orthosis [AFO]) picks up the foot and allows it to follow through in the normal heel-toe manner (Figure 9.1).

An AFO also may be designed to decrease spasticity by tilting the foot to a specified angle and keeping it from turning in or out (inverting or everting). Its proper use decreases fatigue while increasing stability. To provide optimal support, such orthoses must be fitted by a specialist called an *orthotist.* AFOs have been improved in the past few years so that they can be hinged and placed at virtually any appropriate angle. The newer AFOs are stronger and more helpful than previous types.

Modern computer sensing has allowed for the development of battery-operated stimulating devices that may pick up the foot without the more cumbersome bracing. The WalkAide and the

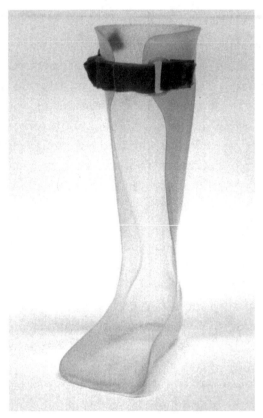

FIGURE 9.1   A rigid polypropylene AFO.

Bioness are examples of these. To utilize these devices, it is important to have enough hip strength to elevate the leg to allow the foot to clear when stimulated. For the appropriate person, these devices are very helpful. They really should be tried under professional supervision before being selected as the device of choice.

You may need a metal brace that fits outside the shoe if you are experiencing a significant increase in tone at the ankle, which is perceived as stiffness. The brace is a spring-loaded device that keeps the toe from dropping. Fortunately, the development of new lightweight materials, including plastics and aluminum, has decreased the need to use the more cumbersome heavy metal (Klenzak™) braces.

If your hip muscles also are weak, you will swing your leg out in front to allow the foot to clear the ground. To maintain stability while doing this, the knee often is forced back farther than it should be, resulting in a condition termed *hyperextension*. This movement puts significant stress on your knee. After a while it will begin to hurt and may become swollen from arthritis. To prevent this condition from developing, a device called a *Swedish hyperextension cage* may be fashioned to prevent the knee from snapping back. A custom-made knee brace may be necessary if the knee cage cannot be fitted properly.

With the aid of such devices, walking with less fatigue may again become realistic. However, if balance also is a problem, another assistive device may be needed such as a cane. Braces, canes, and crutches should be regarded as "tools" in the same way that a hammer or a drill is a carpenter's tool. It is wrong to think that you are "giving in" by using a cane or a brace. If a carpenter wants to drill a hole, he must use the proper drill or the hole will be wrong. A person with impaired mobility who does not use the right tool cannot accomplish the job of walking. Although it may be difficult at first, try not to have negative emotional feelings about using assistive devices. They simply are tools to improve mobility.

A cane usually is carried in the hand *opposite* the weak leg. The activity of walking is reciprocal; that is, the left hand goes forward with the right foot, and vice versa. When a person walks with a cane, the cane should precede or accompany the weak leg. Walking with a cane held on the weak side may cause a noticeable limp.

If weakness is pronounced in both legs, two canes may be needed. The same reciprocal pattern applies: the left foot and right hand go forward together; the right foot and left hand go together. Walking in this fashion is slower, but there always are three points on the ground to provide increased balance and stability.

When climbing stairs, the saying that applies is: "up with the good, down with the bad." Step up first with the strong leg when climbing stairs, and step down first with the weak leg when descending. This pattern makes the strong leg do all the work of lifting and lowering. Again, the cane should accompany or precede the weak leg. Use a railing for support whenever possible. If a railing is on the same side as the cane, merely shift the cane to the other hand and use the stair-walking pattern described.

If balance and weakness are more severe, it may be necessary to use forearm (Lofstrand™) crutches. These crutches provide greater stability than a standard cane, and their use does not require as much strength in the upper extremities. The patterns described for walking with a cane apply equally to walking with the aid of forearm crutches.

A walker may be the proper assistive tool if your balance is especially poor. The usual pattern to be used is as follows: walker forward at arms' length, weak leg, then strong leg. Take normal-sized steps, and avoid stepping past the front of the walker. Walkers come in many varieties. If your gait needs maximum stability, it is best to use a walker without wheels. Some of the newer types have larger wheels as well as seats. They can move very smoothly and allow you to take rest periods by locking the brakes and sitting.

To measure the proper height for all assistive devices, place the device 6 inches away from the side of the foot, and adjust the handles so that the elbow is bent approximately 25 degrees. As with any specialized tool, it is important to have the right tool, to have it fitted properly, and to know how to use it correctly. An experienced physical therapist should be helpful in ensuring a proper fit.

If walking is still extremely difficult or impossible despite the selection of excellent devices, a wheelchair may be your correct choice. You should not resist using a wheelchair; try to view it simply another mobility tool. Selecting from the many types of wheelchairs available depends on many factors, including your size and weight, strength, and level of energy. A standard manual wheelchair often does not offer people with MS sufficient independence because of the fatigue that is generated by operating the chair and the coordination that is necessary to control it.

Three-wheeled motorized scooters are a boon for people with MS because they do not carry the negative stigma with which regular wheelchairs may be inappropriately perceived (Figure 9.2). Although scooters are extremely useful, they are best used by people who have retained some means of walking, because their seating systems are not designed for sitting all day. Those who do not possess the ambulatory skills necessary to use a three-wheeler appropriately may achieve independence with one of the newer, lightweight motorized wheelchairs (Figure 9.3). It is ironic that Medicare and many insurance companies have decided that these chairs should only be used if a person is not ambulatory when they are medically most appropriate for those who possess some ambulatory skills but not efficient ones.

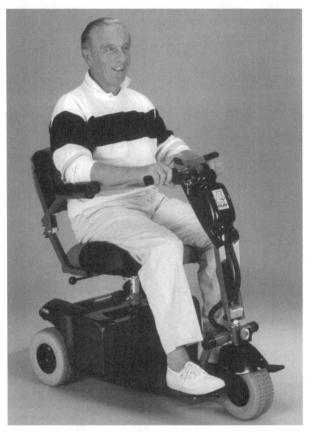

FIGURE **9.2** Lightweight three-wheeled scooter with tiller steering and hand brake. (Courtesy of Bruno Incorporated.)

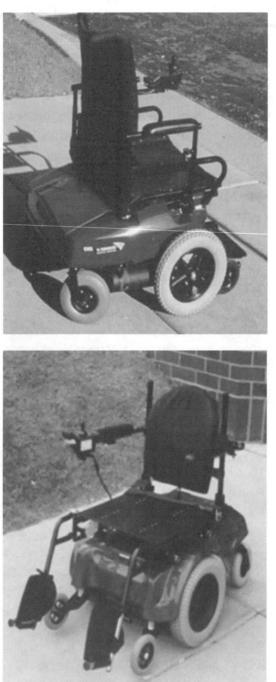

FIGURE 9.3   Lightweight motorized wheelchairs.

The key to choosing a chair or a scooter is *independence*. The proper device should be selected to regain control and independence in the environment. Again, help from a physical therapist, occupational therapist, or a physician who understands the use of the chair is necessary to select the most appropriate one.

There is no reason not to be mobile in today's world. The right assistive device coupled with the right attitude can make all the difference. You must remember that the idea is to get where you want to go. It really does not matter how you get there.

If you need an assistive device to maintain your mobility, transportation by car, bus, van, or other means should accommodate the device. You will need proper consultation for van lifts, and it is essential to learn about local public transportation that will accommodate the devices. Working toward accessibility is in everyone's best interest and should be encouraged in every way that is appropriate to your living situation.

TRANSFERS

When mobility is impaired and the use of a wheelchair is practical, it is essential that you be able to safely transfer in and out of the chair. There are many transfer techniques, including the pivot transfer, the transfer board transfer, and the Hoyer transfer (see Appendix C).

As with all devices, the feelings about their use must be mastered. These devices provide an opportunity for mobility—they are friends, not enemies. The goal must be to learn how to use them and how to transfer safely.

Chapter

10

PRESSURE SORES

Decubiti, also called *pressure sores* or *decubitus ulcers*, are breaks in the skin caused by too much pressure over a period of time. They are only an occasional problem in people with MS, but they are considered a medical emergency when they do occur. If they are managed well when they first develop, they usually resolve without problem; if they are left to increase in size, they may become life-threatening. *The best way to treat a decubitus is to prevent it in the first place.* That means watching for pressure areas (reddened and inflamed) and getting off of them.

Decubiti most commonly occur on the buttocks and other areas that are in constant contact with the surface of a bed or wheelchair. A person with decreased skin sensation does not perceive the discomfort that normally would indicate that he or she has been in one position for too long. Pressure sores frequently appear quietly, with little or no pain, and continue to enlarge, resulting in large holes in the skin that gradually expand into the underlying muscle. Additional factors that may contribute to this process include inadequate nutrition, dependency on certain medications, stool or urine incontinence, and a lack of education regarding prevention.

When pressure is applied to an area of skin over a bony prominence, blood flow to the area is obstructed. The body produces a rebound response of redness and heat when the pressure is relieved, and the skin and muscle below can recover if the pressure does not persist. This is called *healing by first or primary intention.* People with MS should know how to avoid stressing the skin to the point that it cannot recover. Several factors affect wound healing, including age, the presence of other medical problems, and nutritional state.

To repeat: the key to managing decubiti is to avoid them! Avoidance means transferring weight off contact areas at frequent intervals without using pressure, shear, or friction to accomplish the move. It means using proper equipment to disperse the weight of the body over larger surface areas, such as foam pillows, air mattresses, water mattresses, and gels. Foam rubber pads and sheepskins placed under pressure areas such as the sacrum (tail area) and heels aid in dispersing pressure during movement. These "tools," plus proper positioning, relieve shear and friction. The skin must be frequently and carefully examined for areas of pressure and breakdown.

The key to managing pressure sores is to avoid them!

For the bedridden person, a special mattress that takes pressure off the stressed areas may replace the standard bed. It is important to turn once every two hours to avoid continuing pressure to any one area.

Immediate attention is essential if an ulcerated area does form. No pressure should be applied to the area. The good skin around the affected area must be preserved and toughened. Special "skin-like" bandages may be applied. Cleaning the area (debridement) may be necessary and should be performed by someone who is trained in this technique.

If all else fails, surgical closure of the wound may be necessary. Surgery allows for *healing by secondary intention.* The ulcer cavity (opening) with its surrounding scar tissue must be completely removed, the bony edge removed, and the wound covered with healthy skin.

Proper postsurgical management is critical for a favorable outcome. It should be obvious that care must be taken not to irritate the wound until it has healed. Further attention to prevention is even more important after the wound has healed because the area remains vulnerable to reinjury.

If careful attention is paid to the preventive measures described here, the chances of a pressure sore forming will be minimized. *Prevention is the best strategy.*

11

BLADDER SYMPTOMS

Many people with MS experience difficulties with bladder control and urination at some point during the course of the disease. Bladder symptoms usually can be controlled with medication or other approaches that minimize any changes in daily activities and lifestyle.

THE URINARY SYSTEM AND ITS CONTROL

Figure 11.1 shows the urinary system, the main function of which is to collect and eliminate bodily wastes in the form of urine. The urinary system includes:

- The kidneys, which filter the blood to remove waste products and produce urine at a rate of approximately one ounce (30 mL) per hour
- The bladder, a muscular sac that stretches to store the urine until it is emptied by urination, a process referred to as voiding
- The urethra, a hollow tube through which urine passes from the body when voiding occurs

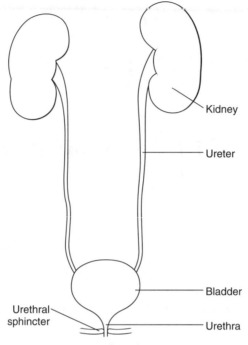

Kidney

Ureter

Bladder

Urethral sphincter

Urethra

FIGURE 11.1   The urinary system.

- The urethral sphincter, a valvelike muscle that opens and closes to control whether urine remains in the bladder or is voided

When 6 to 8 ounces (180–240 mL) of urine is present in the bladder, it becomes sufficiently stretched to stimulate nerve endings located in its wall. These nerves send a signal of fullness to an area in the spinal cord that may be thought of as a "voiding reflex center" (Figure 11.2). This center in turn sends the signal on to the brain, and you become aware of the need to urinate. The brain then signals the spinal center, which sends two signals, one to the bladder telling it to contract and a second to the urethral sphincter muscle telling it to relax. This combination of a contracted bladder and a relaxed sphincter permits urine to flow from the bladder.

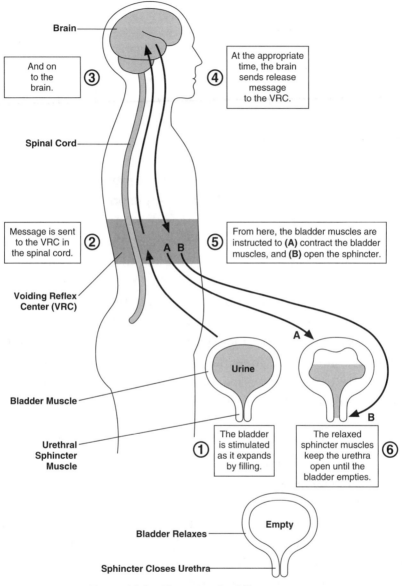

FIGURE 11.2   The normal voiding process.

BLADDER PROBLEMS ASSOCIATED WITH MULTIPLE SCLEROSIS

The elimination of urine by conscious choice is dependent on the integrity of the spinal cord pathways that connect the brain and the voiding reflex center. The downward command by the brain to "empty" causes relaxation and opening of the sphincter, whereas the command to wait signals the sphincter to remain closed. The pathways between the reflex center and the brain may be damaged or interrupted in MS, producing a variety of problems and/or symptoms. The specific nature of the problem depends on the location of the damage. For example, if the connections between the reflex center and the brain are severely damaged, the reflex center may assume direct control of voiding and automatically stimulate the bladder to empty whenever it fills. The most common bladder problems associated with MS are increased frequency of urination, urgency, dribbling, hesitancy, and incontinence.

Frequency involves an increase in the number of times urination occurs within the day. In some people voiding may occur as often as every 15 to 20 minutes, usually in small amounts each time. The frequency of urination depends on the rate at which urine is formed and the ability of the bladder to store it.

Urgency is the feeling of having to empty the bladder immediately combined with an inability to "hold" urine once the urge to void is felt. People who experience this problem have little time to reach a bathroom.

Dribbling is the leakage of small amounts of urine from the bladder. This may occur as the result of urgency and the inability to retain urine. In some cases a person may only be aware of this problem until damp undergarments are noted.

Hesitancy involves difficulty in beginning to urinate after the urge to void is felt. This symptom may be associated with urgency, so that one is unable to urinate while the urge to do so remains.

Incontinence is an inability to hold urine in the bladder. It may result either from not being able to reach the toilet in time or from being unaware of the need to empty the bladder because of blockage of the pathways between the voiding reflex center and the brain. Despite the ability of the bladder to stretch as it fills, it can hold only a certain amount of urine and empties spontaneously after this limit is reached.

Probably the most common type of bladder problem in MS results from a *small spastic bladder,* sometimes referred to as a "failure-to-store" bladder, which results from demyelination of the spinal cord pathways between the voiding reflex center and the brain (Figure 11.3). Because the pathways to the brain are blocked, bladder emptying no longer is under voluntary control. Voiding then becomes a reflex activity, with messages to "empty" coming only from the spinal center. A small spastic bladder may produce symptoms of increased frequency, urgency, dribbling, and/or incontinence (Table 11.1).

When demyelination occurs in the area of the spinal voiding reflex center, messages cannot be transmitted to or from either the brain or the bladder. A *flaccid* or big bladder results (Figure 11.4). The bladder fills with large amounts of urine, but because the spinal center cannot transmit messages on to the brain, the person is unaware of this fullness. Because the spinal center also cannot transmit messages to the bladder and sphincter, there is very little voluntary or reflex control over urination. The bladder fills and then overfills, producing symptoms of frequency, urgency, dribbling, hesitancy, and incontinence. This situation sometimes is referred to as the "failure-to-empty" bladder.

The third type of bladder dysfunction is the *dyssynergic* or "conflicting" bladder, in which the problem is related to coordination between bladder wall contraction and sphincter relaxation (Figure 11.5) rather than with the size of the bladder. In the dyssynergic bladder, either (1) the bladder wall contracts while the sphincter remains closed, resulting in a sense of urgency followed by hesitancy in beginning to void, or (2) the bladder wall relaxes while the sphincter remains open, resulting in dribbling of urine or incontinence. This lack of coordination between the bladder wall

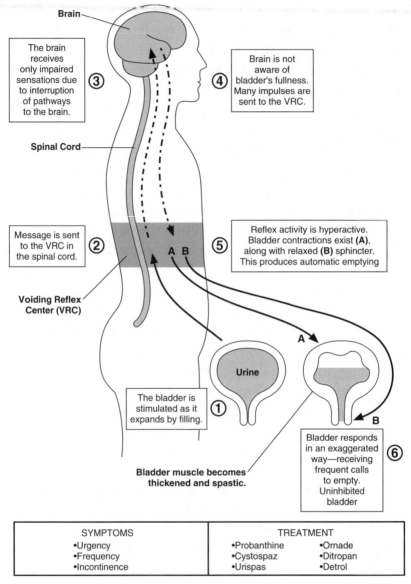

Brain

The brain receives only impaired sensations due to interruption of pathways to the brain. ③

Brain is not aware of bladder's fullness. Many impulses are sent to the VRC. ④

Spinal Cord

Message is sent to the VRC in the spinal cord. ②

Reflex activity is hyperactive. Bladder contractions exist **(A)**, along with relaxed **(B)** sphincter. This produces automatic emptying ⑤

A B

Voiding Reflex Center (VRC)

A

Urine

The bladder is stimulated as it expands by filling. ①

B

Bladder responds in an exaggerated way—receiving frequent calls to empty. Uninhibited bladder ⑥

Bladder muscle becomes thickened and spastic.

SYMPTOMS	TREATMENT	
•Urgency	•Probanthine	•Ornade
•Frequency	•Cystospaz	•Ditropan
•Incontinence	•Urispas	•Detrol

FIGURE 11.3   Spastic "small" bladder.

TABLE 11.1   Types of Bladder Dysfunction

Problem	Symptoms	Treatment
Small, spastic bladder (failure to store)	Increased frequency, urgency, dribbling, and/or incontinence	Oxybutynin (Ditropan®, Ditropan XL®) Hyoscyamine (Levsinex®, Levbid®) Tolterodine tartrate (Detrol®) Flavoxate HCl (Urispas®) Imipramine (Tofranil®) Antihistamines Solfenacin (Vesicare®) Tolterodine tartrate LA (Detrol LA®) Trospium CL (Sanctura®) Darifenacin (Enablex®) Mirebegron (Mybetriq®)
Flaccid (big) bladder (failure to empty)	Frequency, urgency, dribbling, hesitancy, incontinence	Urecholine (Duvoid®) Valsava manuever Credé technique Intermittent self-catheterization
Dyssynergic bladder (conflicting)	EITHER urgency followed by hesitation in beginning to void; OR dribbling or incontinence	Phenoxybenzamine (Dibenzyline®) Terazosin (Hytrin®) Alpha blockers

and the sphincter is frequently seen in combination with either the spastic or the flaccid bladder.

It is important to remember that the bladder does not make urine—urine is made by the kidneys. Disease of the kidneys is not a routine complication of MS. It only occurs if infection of the bladder is uncontrolled and is surprisingly uncommon in MS, which makes the routine kidney X-ray (intravenous pyelogram [IVP]) for the most

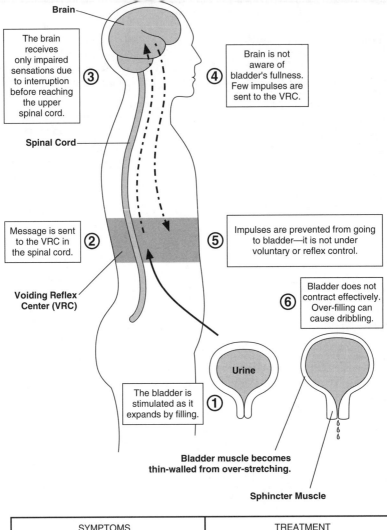

FIGURE 11.4   Flaccid "big" bladder.

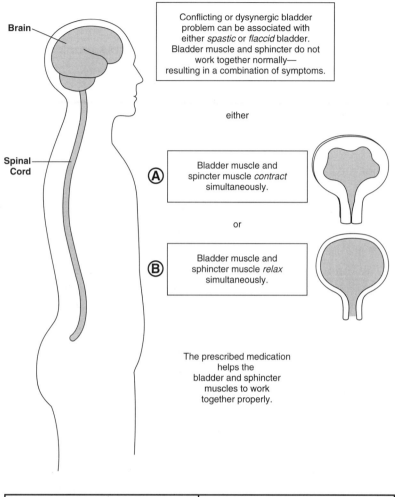

Brain

Conflicting or dysynergic bladder problem can be associated with either *spastic* or *flaccid* bladder. Bladder muscle and sphincter do not work together normally—resulting in a combination of symptoms.

either

Spinal Cord

Ⓐ Bladder muscle and spincter muscle *contract* simultaneously.

or

Ⓑ Bladder muscle and sphincter muscle *relax* simultaneously.

The prescribed medication helps the bladder and sphincter muscles to work together properly.

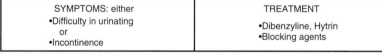

SYMPTOMS: either	TREATMENT
•Difficulty in urinating or •Incontinence	•Dibenzyline, Hytrin •Blocking agents

FIGURE 11.5 Conflicting bladder.

part unnecessary. However, the risk of urine backing up from the bladder toward the kidney is increased in a man with a dyssynergic bladder (women usually do not experience this problem because the pressures within the female bladder are lower). This potential problem must be carefully managed by a physician.

MANAGEMENT OF BLADDER PROBLEMS

Bladder problems often may be managed with medications and/ or other approaches. To determine the most appropriate mode of treatment, it first is necessary to distinguish between the spastic (failure to store), flaccid (failure to empty), and dyssynergic bladder. This is easily done by carefully recording the frequency of urination and the amounts of fluid urinated over a 48-hour period, followed by determining how much urine remains in the bladder after void- ing. Your doctor will measure the amount of this "residual" urine by inserting a catheter into the bladder or by ultrasound technology after urination; a residual of less than 5 ounces (150 mL) indicates either a normal bladder or a small spastic bladder, whereas a larger amount indicates a flaccid bladder.

The small spastic bladder is best treated with medications that "slow" the bladder by decreasing transmission in the nerves to the bladder that cause it to empty. These include oxybutynin (Ditro- pan®, Ditropan XL®, Oxytrol patch®), tolterodine tartrate (Detrol®, Detrol LA®), hyoscyamine (Levsinex®, Levbid®, Cystospaz®), fla- voxate hydrochloride (Urispas®), imipramine (Tofranil®), solfena- cin (Vesicare®), tolterodine tartrate LA (Detrol LA®), trospium CL (Sanctura®), darifenacin (Enablex®), mirabegron (Myrbetriq®), and several medications that are used for the "runny" nose of a cold. These medications lengthen the intervals between urination and decrease urgency, thus allowing for more time to reach the bath- room and avoiding dribbling and incontinence.

Onabotulinumtoxin A (Botox®) can be injected into the bladder wall and the sphincter. This decreases the muscle tone (strength) and may allow for increased urine retention. This treatment is becoming more popular and is now approved by the FDA. It needs to be repeated about every three months as it wears off. An experienced urologist or gynecologist performs this procedure.

Physical therapists have developed not only exercises but also biofeedback techniques that enable people with overactive bladders as a result of MS to learn how to decrease the stimulation of the bladder by using learned sensing in the body. These techniques, when mastered, may result in decreased medication use.

Treatment of the flaccid bladder is not as simple, and management frequently relies on alternative techniques for bladder emptying rather than on medication. One common method that facilitates more complete bladder emptying is the *Credé technique* of bladder massage. This technique involves applying downward pressure to the lower abdomen with both hands while bearing down after as much urine as possible has been voided naturally; it is necessary for men to sit while using the technique. This technique should not be used in the dyssynergic bladder because the urine may back up into the kidneys. This mainly is a problem in men because pressure is much lower in the female bladder.

If the bladder cannot be emptied sufficiently by the Credé technique, *intermittent self-catheterization* may be used for more complete bladder emptying. A small tube, or *catheter,* is inserted through the urethra into the bladder to allow the urine to drain out. This may seem rather complicated, but actually it is simple to learn and it poses no risk. It allows a person to empty the bladder at planned intervals, thus avoiding dribbling or incontinence. The frequency of self-catheterization varies from person to person but generally need not be done more frequently than every four to six hours. Medications such as oxybutynin frequently are used in conjunction with self-catheterization to allow the bladder to fill more completely and to decrease the need to urinate between catheterizations. To do this properly there should be decent coordination in the hands and reasonable sensation in the fingers. Without that it is not practical to embark on this trail even if the bladder is appropriate for it. To ask a relative to do this technique on a regular basis is usually a major mistake because the relationship at a personal level almost always changes negatively because of the removal of privacy and social issues.

There is a surgical procedure in which the bladder is enlarged by splicing a piece of the colon to it. Another piece of intestine (often the appendix) is attached to this enlarged bladder and brought to the outside of the body through the belly button (umbilicus). This allows for the intermittent catheter to be inserted in a very visible location and allows performance despite some disabilities. The surgery is not minor and must be thought out and performed by an experienced urologist.

As mentioned previously, conflict or dyssynergia often is combined with either a spastic bladder or a flaccid bladder. Initial treatment based on the 48-hour diary is aimed at either spasticity or flaccidity; if the previously described techniques do not provide adequate control, it becomes apparent that the bladder wall and the sphincter are not functioning in a coordinated fashion. Occasionally, formal testing with a "bladder analysis machine" (cystometer) is needed to accurately pinpoint the source of the problem. The problem may be helped by the addition of an alpha blocker to the treatment regimen. Most alpha blockers were developed to aid in the treatment of high blood pressure, but they also help the bladder work in a more coordinated manner. Phenoxybenzamine (Dibenzyline®), clonidine, and terazosin (Hytrin®) are alpha blockers that improve coordination and increase bladder control.

Problems with incontinence may occur mainly at night during sleep. One approach to this problem involves the use of a medication named DDAVP® (desmopressin), a hormone that slows the production of urine by the kidneys. DDAVP comes in many forms, but the most practical form is now a pill. One or two pills decrease urine formation during the night and decrease the chances of a wet bed. This helps one to get a good night's sleep, which may decrease morning fatigue. The body eliminates the stored fluid during the daytime, so the person needs to be able to control his or her bladder during the day. DDAVP is very expensive.

If a bladder problem cannot be controlled with medication and/or intermittent self-catheterization, continuous (chronic) catheterization may become necessary. This is done with a permanent *Foley catheter.* This type of catheter is used only when absolutely necessary because it is associated with an increased incidence of urinary tract infection (UTI). The quality of life may be increased significantly by a Foley catheter as one spends less time worrying about the bladder and more time with appropriate activities. An indwelling Foley catheter may irritate the bladder wall, and bladder stones may form in response to this irritation. Bladder stones may increase the likelihood of infection and decrease urinary flow. The stones usually are removed by a fairly simple surgical procedure called a *cystoscopy,* which is performed through a "scope" that the urologist uses to look into the bladder.

Medtronic has developed a bladder stimulator (InterStim®) which is an implantable neurostimulator carrying electrical impulses through a wire into the nerves controlling the pelvic wall. This has not been well studied in MS and should be reserved for difficult situations evaluated by a urologist trained in neurourology. When a stimulator is implanted, follow-up MRI's looking at MS progress are limited because the magnet of the MRI heats the wires to potentially burning temperatures.

With chronic, significant infections, the bladder wall may become so damaged that the infection cannot be cleared and the bladder must be bypassed or diverted. A piece of intestine is used to divert the urine to a bag on the body like a colostomy. This procedure is reserved for extreme situations, but it does permit infection to be controlled more easily.

A condom-type catheter also may be used by men. The penis must be of sufficient size that the condom has enough area to adhere to the shaft. Because this area is damp and mechanical stress is involved, care must be taken not to let ulcers develop on the penis. Unfortunately, female condom catheters are not sufficiently reliable to be used on a regular basis.

URINARY TRACT (BLADDER) INFECTION

Urinary tract infection (UTI) is an example of a "secondary problem" in MS. UTI is not a direct result of the demyelination process, but occurs as the result of (secondary to) the retention of urine in the bladder. Mild infection may result only in increased frequency and urgency of urination, whereas severe infection produces fever and generalized illness.

The incidence of UTI is higher than normal in (1) those who have a flaccid bladder, because bacteria may grow in the retained urine, (2) those who need to perform intermittent self-catheterization, and (3) those who have an indwelling Foley catheter, which may provide bacteria with a direct route into the bladder. Women generally are at higher risk for the development of bladder infection than men. The diagnosis of a UTI is made by a *urine culture,* in which urine is collected in a sterile fashion and tested for the presence of bacteria. The presence of bacteria in the urine does not necessarily mean that there is an infection that requires treatment. Many people with MS have what is described as "asymptomatic bacteriuria," especially if they have an indwelling Foley catheter. If the person is asymptomatic, without pain, fever, or other signs of the spread of infection, it is appropriate simply to watch the process.

Other symptoms of a UTI may include frequent urination, urgency, burning, or discomfort when urinating, fever, or foul-smelling urine accompanied by the presence of blood or mucus. Because some of these symptoms are similar to symptoms frequently experienced by an individual with MS, treatment should not be started until the presence of infection has been confirmed. Generally, infection is suspected when symptoms occur suddenly or if fever is present. A urine specimen is cultured in the laboratory to confirm that bacteria are present before treatment is initiated with an antibiotic specific for the organism causing the infection; the antibiotic generally is taken for 7 to 10 days. New antibiotics are being developed constantly, and they have been very helpful in managing severe bladder infection.

Bladder infection may largely be prevented by complete bladder emptying, using self-catheterization techniques if necessary.

> *Prevention is the key to avoiding bladder infections.*

Bacterial growth is prevented or retarded when the urine is acidic, which is best achieved by taking high doses of vitamin C. A person who has a history of UTI may be helped by substances that suppress the growth of bacteria in the urine and low doses of antibiotics, usually sulfa or nitrofurantoin. Prevention is the key to avoiding bladder infections.

- Urination should be frequent and complete, and holding urine in the bladder for long periods should be avoided.
- Women should be careful to wipe from front to back, especially after a bowel movement, and should avoid undergarments that are made of synthetic materials, which tend to trap moisture. Women who have recurrent infections should empty the bladder both before and after intercourse.
- Adequate amounts of fluid should be taken to keep the bladder "flushed." Generally six to eight glasses per day is sufficient.
- Those who are prone to the development of bladder infection should take up to 1000 mg of vitamin C four times each day to make their urine more acidic, because higher acidity inhibits bacterial growth.

People who have an indwelling Foley catheter should be especially careful to keep the catheter, tubing, and drainage bag as clean as possible. The catheter should be changed at least once a month, using proper sterile technique.

Urinary tract infection may pose a serious threat to health if it is not properly treated, so it is very important to seek medical attention if symptoms occur.

UTI may pose a serious threat to health if it is not properly treated, so it is very important to seek medical attention if symptoms occur.

When a UTI does occur, the key to treatment is the use of an appropriate antibiotic, as indicated by the results of the urine culture and a related test for the antibiotic sensitivity of the infecting organism. It is important that this medication be taken as directed *for the complete time period indicated* to ensure that all the invading bacteria are destroyed. It is a mistake to stop taking an antibiotic if you are feeling better because not all the bacteria may have been destroyed; the remaining bacteria will reinvade and cause further problems.

BLADDER SPASMS

The bladder sometimes contracts involuntarily. The result often is pain and a squirt of urine that may lead to total emptying of the bladder. If a catheter is in place, the urine will leak out around it. This is a bladder spasm. The medications used for leg spasms (see Chapter 5) often are helpful in this event, as are the medications used for the small, spastic bladder.

INCONTINENCE PADS

The variety of incontinence devices and pads has multiplied during the last decade. There are many kinds of adult incontinence devices and diapers. When choosing one of these products, look for a pad or diaper that prevents skin irritation and offensive odor, and is comfortable. It is beyond the scope of this chapter to discuss this topic in detail, but improvements are occurring constantly and must be assessed accordingly.

C h a p t e r

12

Bowel Symptoms

As with the urinary tract, many people with MS have some degree of bowel complication at some point during the course of the disease. These difficulties may be effectively managed with medications and other treatments.

The Gastrointestinal Tract and Its Control

The gastrointestinal (GI) tract is a hollow, muscular tube that extends from the mouth to the anus and is responsible for the digestion and absorption of food followed by elimination of the waste products of the digestion process.

The *stomach* primarily acts as a storage chamber and is the first site of major digestive processes. It slowly passes food to the *small intestine*, which in turn sends it to the *large intestine* by a propulsive movement.

The large intestine is approximately five feet long and is divided into four sections: the ascending, transverse, descending, and sigmoid colon. In the sigmoid colon, stool is concentrated into a solid mass by the absorption of much of the fluid that is present in other areas of the tract. The reflex process that leads to a bowel movement (defecation) occurs when stool moves from the sigmoid colon into the rectum, the last four to six inches of the tract.

The rectum usually remains empty until just before and during defecation, when stool enters it either as a result of a mass propulsive movement or by voluntary contraction of the abdominal muscles. In a manner similar to what happens when the bladder initiates urination, filling of the rectum with stool causes nerve endings in the rectal wall to transmit a message of fullness to an area of the spinal cord that is involved in bowel function. As stool leaves the rectum, it passes through the *anal canal*, which contains the *internal* and *external sphincter* muscles. The sphincters, ring-shaped muscles that control the opening and closing of the passageway from the rectum, normally are contracted to prevent leakage. The internal sphincter is under the control of the spinal cord; its relaxation is what is termed an involuntary reflex because it is not under conscious control, and its relaxation depends only on stretching of the rectal wall by stool. In contrast, the external sphincter is under the joint control of the spinal cord and the brain, so that a bowel movement may be consciously delayed by constricting the anus if the time is not appropriate for a bowel movement. The most common bowel problems associated with MS are constipation, diarrhea, and incontinence.

CONSTIPATION

Constipation is defined as the infrequent or difficult elimination of stool. It is by far the most common bowel problem associated with MS and may result from one or several problems that are direct or indirect consequences of the disease.

- Demyelination in the brain and/or spinal cord may interfere with the nerve transmission that is necessary for normal defecation in a manner similar to that described in Chapter 10. A slower-than-normal passage of stool through the bowel results in more water being removed from it than is normal, which results in hard, constipating stool.

- A person with MS may limit fluid intake because of bladder difficulties. If fluid intake is insufficient to allow the body to meet its basic needs, more water will be absorbed as the stool passes through the colon, which also produces hard, compacted stool that is difficult to pass.
- Weakness, spasticity, or fatigue may significantly limit physical activity, which in turn slows bowel activity and the movement of stool through the GI tract; again, excessive amounts of water will be absorbed from the stool, causing it to harden and become difficult to pass.

Some of the medications taken for other problems such as bladder frequency or depression also may slow the bowel.

THE DEVELOPMENT OF GOOD BOWEL HABITS: DIETARY MANAGEMENT

Good eating habits are important to achieving good bowel control. It is important to have a routine and to eat balanced meals at regular times and in a relaxed atmosphere (Table 12.1). The intake of adequate amounts of liquid (8–12 cups daily) and the addition of fiber to the diet generally alleviates constipation. Dietary fiber is that portion of plant materials that is resistant to digestion; its addition to the diet aids in the formation of softer stool and decreases the amount of time required for stool to pass through the intestinal tract.

TABLE 12.1   Bowel-Habit Management

- Eat a high-fiber diet of balanced meals
- Drink 8 to 12 cups of fluid daily
- Establish a bowel program
- Medications

A high-fiber diet includes raw fruits and vegetables, nuts and seeds, and whole grain breads and cereals such as cornmeal, cracked and whole wheat, barley, graham, wild and brown rice, and bran (one of the most concentrated sources of dietary fiber).

To increase the amount of fiber in your diet, your daily intake should include:

- One serving of fruit (with the skin left on) or vegetable, served cooked, raw, or dried
- One-half to one serving of fruit juice
- One-half to one serving of whole wheat or rye bread
- One serving of bran (one tablespoon), bran cereal, shredded wheat, nuts or seeds; raw bran may be eaten plain; mixed with cereal, applesauce, soups, yogurt, or casseroles; or added to flour in cooking or baking

Incorporating bran and other high-fiber foods into the diet too quickly may produce gas, distention, and occasionally diarrhea. These effects may be eliminated or lessened substantially if high-fiber foods are incorporated in small amounts and then gradually increased.

ESTABLISHING A BOWEL PROGRAM

Because decreased sensation in the rectal area in MS may decrease perception of the need to have a bowel movement, stool may remain in the rectum and become hard and constipating. Although this and other factors may lead to constipation becoming a significant problem, it is manageable with a commitment to following an established elimination schedule, timing of meals, fluid intake, and the use of medications if necessary. The first step in establishing a bowel program is to select the time that is most convenient to have a bowel movement. Although this may vary depending on your job commitments, family routines, and other daily activities, the most effective time to have a bowel movement is shortly after a meal because there normally is a greater movement of contents through the bowel at that time. With this in mind, 15 to 30 minutes of uninterrupted time in which to have a bowel movement should be scheduled.

After a convenient time has been selected, it is important to adhere to this routine on a daily basis, whether or not you feel an urge to defecate. Drinking a cup of warm liquid, such as coffee, tea, or water, frequently facilitates the process. Although this schedule initially may produce little result, it is imperative that the routine be adhered to if a successful bowel program is to be established.

Medications

Medications may be needed if constipation cannot be corrected by changing the diet, increasing fluid intake, and/or establishing a routine. To determine the most appropriate medication, the reason for the constipation must be determined, because it may be caused by lack of bulk, hard stools, or difficulty in expelling stool (Table 12.2). *Bulk formers* may be prescribed if the cause of constipation is inadequate bulk in the diet and stool. These agents add substance to the stool by increasing its bulk and water content. In order to be effective, bulk formers should be taken with one or two glasses of liquid; this combination distends the GI tract, which in turn increases the passage of stool through it. Defecation usually occurs within 12 to 24 hours, although in some cases it may be delayed for up to three days.

TABLE 12.2   Medications for the Management of Constipation

Medication	Indications for Use
Bulk formers	Inadequate bulk in the diet and stool
Stool softeners	Hard stool causes constipation
Laxative (oral stimulant)	Difficulty expelling stool
Suppositories and other rectal Stimulants	In combination with other medications if necessary
Enemeez® mini-enemas	When lubricating stimulation is helpful
Enemas	For occasional use only, to avoid dependency

The daily use of bulk formers is necessary for maximal effectiveness. They are not habit-forming, so frequent use is not a problem.

Common bulk formers include:

- Metamucil®, taken in a dose of 1 to 2 teaspoons daily mixed in a glass of water or juice and followed by an extra glass of fluid. This may be increased to one teaspoon taken two or three times per day if necessary.
- FiberCon®, two tablets, one to four times a day; each dose should be followed by 8 ounces of liquid.
- Citrucel®, one tablespoon, one to three times daily, mixed in 8 ounces of juice or water.
- Fiberall®, available in chewable tablets, wafers, or powder, may be taken one to three times a day with 8 ounces of liquid.

Stool Softeners

If the cause of constipation is hard stool, stool softeners are used to draw increased amounts of water from body tissues into the bowel, thereby decreasing hardness and facilitating elimination. Consistent use is recommended to obtain maximal benefit; as with bulk formers, stool softeners are not habit-forming. They include:

- Colace® (docusate): take one pill every morning and evening.
- Surfak®: take one pill every morning.
- Chronulac® syrup: take one ounce every evening, increasing to one ounce each morning and evening if necessary.

Laxatives (Oral Stimulants)

If difficulty in expelling stool is the cause of constipation, it may be corrected with laxatives, also referred to as oral stimulants. Laxatives provide a chemical irritant to the bowel. Although a number of over-the-counter laxatives are available, care should be taken to avoid the use of harsh laxatives, which may be highly habit-forming. The same results may be obtained by using the following milder laxatives,

> *Care should be taken to avoid the use of harsh laxatives, which may be highly habit-forming.*

which are less harmful to the bowel and induce bowel movements gently, usually overnight or within 8 to 12 hours:

- Peri-Colace®: take one or two capsules at bedtime; increase to two capsules twice a day if necessary.
- Milk of Magnesia®: take 1 ounce at bedtime every other day.
- MiraLax® (telmisartan) is a laxative that can be very effective for problematic constipation.

Suppositories and Other Rectal Stimulants

Rectal stimulants provide both chemical stimulation and localized mechanical stimulation combined with lubrication to promote stool elimination. They may be used either occasionally when necessary or on a routine daily or every-other-day basis in conjunction with other medications already listed. Suppositories generally act within 15 minutes to an hour. They include:

- Glycerin suppositories, which contain no medication and provide rectal stimulation and lubrication for easier passage of stool. Glycerin suppositories are milder and less habit-forming than Dulcolax® and are used to help develop a bowel routine.
- Dulcolax® suppositories, which contain a medication that is absorbed by the lining of the large bowel and stimulates a strong wavelike movement of the rectal muscles that facilitates elimination.
- Enemeez®, which are not traditional enemas but rather lubricating stimulants in an easy-to-administer shell. This preparation is a clean way of administering a helpful medication to stimulate a bowel movement.

Enemas may be considered an occasional treatment for constipation, but *the frequent use of enemas should be avoided* because the bowel may become dependent on them when they are used routinely.

In summary, many medications are available without a prescription for the treatment of constipation, but their indiscriminate use should be avoided. A professional should be consulted to determine which medication or combination of medications is best suited to a specific problem. In attempting to control constipation, it may be necessary to begin a bowel program that includes a number of medications. This may seem rather overwhelming in the beginning, but some medications may be eliminated as a routine is established and bowel movements become more regular. *Consistency is the key to regulating constipation.*

DIARRHEA AND INCONTINENCE

Diarrhea is much less common than constipation in people with MS. However, it may be a significant problem because there may not be adequate warning of an impending attack and incontinence may therefore occur. The probable cause of such diarrhea is a reflex-like activity that results from the short-circuiting in MS, causing frequent emptying even though the bowel is not full.

The key to controlling diarrhea is to make the stool bulkier without producing constipation. Bulk formers such as Metamucil® may be helpful because they absorb water and therefore make the stool firmer. When it is used to treat diarrhea, a bulk former should be taken no more than once a day, and it should not be followed by the recommended extra fluid that is needed when a bulk former is used to treat constipation. In extreme cases, medications that slow the movement of the bowel muscles may be needed to control diarrhea, such as Kaopectate®, Imodium®, or Lomotil®.

Other causes of diarrhea must be considered. A loose stool in a person with MS most often is caused by something other than MS!

Chapter
13

SPEECH DIFFICULTIES

Speech patterns are controlled by many areas of the brain. Depending on the location of demyelinated areas, many alterations of normal speech patterns may occur as the result of MS. Most such alterations affect speech production, resulting in *dysarthria*, or slurred speech, ranging from mild difficulties to severe problems that make comprehension impossible.

Demyelination in the cerebellum, the area of the brain involved with balance, is the primary cause of speech difficulties. Speech generally becomes slow, and fluency is diminished. Words may be slurred, but they usually are understandable. If the tongue, lips, teeth, cheeks, palate, or respiratory muscles become involved, the speech pattern becomes even more slurred (dysarthric). In either case, speech therapy may increase both fluency and speech rhythm. Although exercises are sometimes advocated, they usually are not successful for this type of speech problem. Nevertheless, they may be worth a try.

Oral motor exercises may be used to maintain muscle coordination. The following is a list of exercises that may be done once or twice a day for 20 to 30 minutes with several repetitions:

1. Open and close the mouth slowly several times.
2. Pucker the lips into a big kiss: hold, then relax.
3. Spread the lips into a big smile: hold, then relax.

4. Pucker, hold, smile, hold: repeat this alternating movement.
5. Open the mouth and then try to pucker with the mouth wide open (do not close the jaw): hold, then relax.
6. Close the lips tightly and press together: relax.
7. Close the lips firmly, slurp all the saliva out to the top of the tongue.
8. Open the mouth and stick out the tongue, but be sure the tongue comes straight out of the mouth and does not go off to the side: hold, then relax.
9. Stick out the tongue and move it slowly from corner to corner of the lips; hold in each corner (be sure the tongue actually touches each corner each time), then relax.
10. Stick out the tongue and try to reach the chin with the tongue tip: hold at the farthest point, then relax.
11. Stick out the tongue and try to reach the nose with the tongue tip, but do not use the bottom lip or fingers as a helper: hold as far up as possible, then relax.
12. Stick out the tongue: pretend to lick a sucker, moving the tongue tip from down by the chin up to the nose: go slowly and use as much movement as possible, then relax.
13. Stick out the tongue and pull it back: repeat as many times and as quickly as possible, then rest.
14. Move the tongue from corner to corner as quickly as possible: rest.
15. Move the tongue all around the lips in a circle as quickly and as completely as possible; touch all of both the upper lip, corner, lower lip, corner in a circle; rest.
16. Open and close the mouth as quickly as possible (be sure lips close each time): rest.
17. Say "pa-pa-pa-pa" as quickly as possible without losing the "pa" sound (be sure there is a "p" and an "ah" each time): rest.
18. Say "ta-ta-ta-ta" as quickly and as accurately as possible: rest, then repeat.

19. Say "ka ka ka-ka" as quickly and as accurately as possible: rest, then repeat.
20. Say "pataka, pataka, pataka" (or "buttercup") as quickly and as accurately as possible: rest.

Tremors of the lips, tongue, or jaw also may affect speech by interfering either with breath control for phrasing and loudness or with the ability to voice and pronounce sounds. Speech therapy focuses on increasing the ability to communicate efficiently. It may involve making changes in the rate of speaking or in the phrasing of sentences. Pacing and pausing techniques may be helpful if speech is slurred and rapid. The pausing is used between one or two words. A paceboard initially may be used to assist with this technique. Although it sounds relatively simple, it takes a lot of practice and learning to monitor yourself. Move the fingers along the board for each word produced. Exaggerating (overarticulating) speech sometimes will assist in slowing. Each sound within a word is pronounced, especially the final sounds.

Nonverbal techniques may be used in severe cases of speech intelligibility. These may include the use of a communication board (letter, word, or picture) and a variety of electronic systems. Recently a number of computer-like devices have been developed that fall under what is called "augmentative communication." These include voice synthesizers and microphones that enhance voice loudness. These need to be fit to the specific situation but are very powerful communication devices.

The world of speech has gone high tech!

C h a p t e r

14

SWALLOWING DIFFICULTIES

Dysphagia, or difficulty in swallowing, may be very bothersome in MS. "Swallowing" refers to the passage of food from the mouth into the throat, down the esophagus (food tube), and into the stomach. Swallowing occurs in four stages:

1. The oral preparatory stage involves chewing and preparing the food for swallowing.
2. The oral stage allows the tongue to push the food and move it within the mouth to the back of the mouth.
3. The pharyngeal stage follows and initiates the swallow. The food or liquid is moved into the pharynx (the back of the mouth) and the beginning of the throat.
4. From there begins the esophageal stage, which carries the food into the stomach.

Food may "stick" in the throat, go into the windpipe (trachea), or travel sluggishly and inefficiently, causing coughing, sputtering, and anxiety. Signs of swallowing dysfunction include:

- Gurgling sounds and sounds of congestion
- Spitting or coughing after meals
- An inability to "get the food down"
- Weight loss
- Pneumonia

- Throat clearing
- Choking
- A weak voice

A swallowing evaluation should include a speech pathologist's examination. An "X-ray in motion" (videofluoroscopy) is important to demonstrate the specific location of problems in the swallowing mechanism. In this examination foods and liquids of various consistencies are given while videotaping the swallowing mechanism. After these evaluations, a management plan may be constructed.

The goal of a management plan is to improve nutritional status while making swallowing safe. This may be done by:

- Modifying food textures, because some foods may be swallowed more easily than others. The studies described previously lead to decisions about the texture of food. Sometimes a commercially available thickening agent or gelatin must be added to increase bulk. Milk products may need to be limited because they "stick" in the throat and may be irritating.
- Moistening food with broth, juice, gravy, or fat may allow for a smoother passage.
- Warming or cooling foods may help by stimulating the swallowing reflex.
- Changing the position of the head may be necessary. Tipping the chin down slows the entry of food, especially thin liquids, whereas tilting the head backwards hastens their entry.
- Alternating liquid with solid food prevents sticking in the throat.
- Reducing the size of meals and increasing their frequency so that the appropriate caloric intake is achieved if eating is slow.
- Changing bite size makes a big difference.

Other techniques taught by speech pathologists are important. These include:

- The "power" or "safe" swallow. The person first inhales, then holds his or her breath, which closes the airway so that whatever is being swallowed cannot cause choking. He or she then exhales, swallows again, and exhales yet again.
- Thermal stimulation. The back of the throat is stimulated with a dentist's mirror or something cold, which triggers the swallow reflex.
- Oral motor exercises. These are exercises for the tongue, lips, and soft palate that are designed to make swallowing easier.
- Laryngeal exercises. These involve closing the vocal cords while holding the breath.

Mealtimes are important because they provide social interaction as well as nourishment. It is essential that meals be served at a safe time. If swallowing is a problem, the previously described techniques may be of value. It also is important that the Heimlich maneuver be learned by those who help the person with MS. In extreme cases it may be necessary to have a feeding tube placed directly into the stomach, which may be done under local anesthesia with minimal risk. This alternate nutritional route may help to maintain strength. The person's main nutrition may thus be given without the problems that swallowing presents, with "social chewing" being allowed for special foods.

Chapter

15

VISION

Seeing is very important for all of us, but in MS vision is all too often affected. Many steps are involved in actually seeing an object. The process begins in the eyes. The two major components of effective vision that involve the eye itself are the ability to correctly image what you see and the proper coordination of the muscles that surround the eye and control its movements. Either or both of these can be affected in MS.

Optic or *retrobulbar neuritis* is the term used when the myelinated fibers of the optic nerve are inflamed. If the inflammation can be seen with an ophthalmoscope, it is an optic neuritis. If the inflammation is behind the eye globe, it is termed *retrobulbar* and cannot be seen with the ophthalmoscope. This can be the result of MS or other conditions. The optic nerve is highly myelinated and is an outpocketing of the brain; it is thus very prone to demyelination and inflammation. This results in an acute overall loss of vision. Many studies have shown that vision usually will return whether aggressive treatment is offered or not. However, high-dose steroids will result in more rapid improvement (if it is going to improve). They are often given in form of *high-dose intravenous methylprednisolone*. Oral steroids are often avoided because some studies have shown adverse effects; physicians do not want to take any chances even though these data are not conclusive.

Each person's optic neuritis needs to be looked at individually in terms of treatment and prognosis. In some cases, vision remains imperfect even after inflammation has been reduced. This is especially noticeable at night when lighting is dim, although in normal light colors may appear "washed out." Leaving a light on at night may be helpful. Additionally, there sometimes may be "holes" in the vision, with part of the area one is looking at obscured. This cannot be treated with eyeglasses, which only tend to magnify these areas. It is possible to adjust to the problem over time.

Weakened coordination and strength of the eye muscles produces *double vision*. If this comes on suddenly, it is considered an acute attack and may be treated with steroids. With time, the brain usually learns to compensate for double vision so that images are perceived as normal despite the weakened muscles. *This compensation will not occur if the eye is patched.* Patching should be reserved for reading, driving, or watching television. Prisms placed into eyeglasses may bring images together and provide another relatively simple way to manage this difficult problem.

Jerking eyes may occur in MS; this is called *nystagmus*. MS may be accompanied by various varieties of nystagmus. It usually is more of a nuisance than a major problem. Clonazepam (Klonopin®), memantine (Namenda®), gabapentin (Neurontin®), and other related drugs occasionally decrease nystagmus.

Cataracts (a clouding of the lens of the eye) also may decrease vision in people with MS. Because cortisone promotes the development of cataracts, they often develop at an earlier age than normal in the MS population. Surgical removal of the abnormal lens sometimes brings about a substantial improvement in vision.

As with all symptoms of MS, significant fluctuations in visual symptoms may occur. Visual acuity often falls, and double vision may increase with fatigue, increases in temperature (Uthoff's phenomenon), stress, and infection. Managing these symptoms may help improve vision under those conditions.

Chapter

16

PAIN

Although MS generally is considered to be a painless disease, more than 50% of people with MS find that pain is a problem, and for 10% to 20% it is a significant problem. Pain appears to result from what might be termed *short-circuits* in the tracts that carry sensory impulses between the brain and the spinal cord.

Trigeminal neuralgia occasionally is seen in individuals with MS. This severe, stabbing facial pain usually is treated with carbamazepine (Tegretol®), which appears to "calm" some of the short-circuiting in the sensory areas. To avoid its primary side effect of sleepiness, the medication initially is given at low doses and slowly increased to a point at which it adequately controls the pain. Other medications that may be used to control trigeminal neuralgia include phenytoin (Dilantin®), which has an action that is similar to but milder than that of carbamazepine; baclofen, which most commonly is used for spasticity; and Cytotec®, a medication that is taken for gastric distress. Newer anticonvulsants (used for epilepsy) that also can decrease neuralgic pain include gabapentin (Neurontin®), pregabalin (Lyrica®), oxcarbazepine (Trileptal®), lamotrigine (Lamictal®), levetiracetam (Keppra®), and tiagabine HCl (Gabitril®).

If medications fail to control pain, a surgical procedure may be performed to eliminate the pain, leaving a much less disturbing numbness in its place. This procedure, called *percutaneous rhizotomy,* is performed under local anesthesia with laser technology. Although it is not the first line of therapy, it is viable as a backup. The Gamma Knife is now also used to surgically ablate the nerve without actually cutting.

Occasionally, an unusual "electrical" sensation is felt down the spine and into the legs when the neck is moved. This is a momentary sensation, called *Lhermitte's sign,* which usually is surprising and disturbing. It is a signal of loss of myelin within the spinal cord in the neck region. It has no significance in terms of predicting the course of MS.

Some will feel a "hug"-like sensation across the abdomen (belly). This has been described as the "MS Hug" and for some is very disturbing. Typically it is not a situation for panic but understanding that sensory sensations come and go in MS and are not unusual.

The predominant type of pain seen in MS is a burning, toothache-type pain that occurs most commonly in the extremities, although it also may occur on the trunk. The same medications that are used for trigeminal neuralgia are used for these burning "dysesthesias," but they appear to be less effective than they are for this burning pain. An antiepileptic drug, gabapentin (Neurontin®), has become a useful treatment for this type of discomfort. In doses of 1800 to 2400 mg per day, gabapentin significantly lessens the pain with relatively minimal side effects. Neurontin® has a very short half-life of four hours, which means that half of it is gone every four hours. From a practical point of view this means that the medication usually must be taken at least four times a day. It also means that enough must be taken to be effective. That amount is highly variable. Some people with MS have found that antipain cream (Zostrix®, or capsaic acid) may be helpful. Pregabalin (Lyrica®) and other similar antiseizure medications are often quite effective in decreasing neuropathic pain.

Electrical stimulation (transcutaneous nerve stimulation, or TNS) applied over the area of pain occasionally provides relief. However, it frequently has the opposite effect and therefore is not often recommended. Acupuncture may be helpful for the pain associated with MS, but, unfortunately, even in the best of hands it usually fails over the long term.

Mood-altering drugs such as tranquilizers and antidepressants may be effective in some cases because they alter the interpretation of the message of pain. Several such drugs are available, and some relief may be provided with careful manipulation of the type and dose. Amitriptyline (Elavil®) is the best known of these medications.

Marijuana is legal for medical purposes in some states and is often recommended for MS pain with some success. Please see Chapter 5 on spasticity for the issues surrounding marijuana use that make it something that needs to be discussed on an individual basis in the geographic areas in which it is legally used.

Additionally, biofeedback, meditation, and similar techniques may be of help in specific circumstances. Because pain is a symptom that clearly increases in severity when it is dwelt on, a concerted effort to treat the reaction to pain is an important part of the overall treatment plan.

What is clear is that standard pain medications, including aspirin, codeine, and narcotic analgesics are not effective because the source of pain is not the same as that of the pain that occurs with injury. *Pain medications are therefore to be avoided. They are not only ineffective, but also addictive.*

Centralized pain clinics usually staffed by anesthesiologists (physicians who put people to sleep during surgery) or physiatrists (rehab-trained physicians) have become very popular. They vary a great deal as to philosophy. What is important for those with MS pain to understand is that simply taking narcotics will not improve the situation over the long run. There may be some short-term gains but lots of potential problems later, so it is important to know the philosophy of the pain clinic before beginning therapy there.

Although "MS pain" may be severe and bothersome, it usually does not lead to decreased ambulation and is not predictive of a poor prognosis. In fact, those who have these unusual sensations as the major feature of MS tend to do better than average in movement activities.

Severe pain can result from spasticity and spasms. Management strategies for these are discussed in Chapter 5.

Low back pain is one of the most common symptoms treated by the neurologist, and it therefore is not unexpected that it also is relatively common in people with MS. MS in itself rarely causes low back pain; it more commonly is the result of a pinched nerve or another problem. This situation occurs fairly frequently because of abnormal posture or an unusual MS-related walking pattern, which places stress on the discs of the spine (pad-like structures that cushion the areas between the vertebrae). This stress may cause "slippage" of the discs, compressing one or more of the nerves as they leave the spinal cord and resulting in pain in the part of the body that is innervated by these nerves. Obviously, heavy lifting and inappropriate turning and bending compound the problem. These movements irritate the spinal nerves, causing the muscles on the side of the spinal column (the paraspinal muscles) to go into spasm; it is this spasm that causes low back pain. If a spinal nerve is significantly irritated, the pain may extend down to the muscles in the leg that are served (innervated) by that nerve.

If the problem is one of poor walking posture, the pattern should be corrected; if spasticity contributes to the problem, it must be lessened. Local back care with heat, massage, and ultrasound waves frequently are helpful, and exercises designed to relieve back muscle spasm may be recommended. Physical therapists and chiropractors who are sensitive to the problems associated with MS may speed healing. Drugs designed to relieve back spasms also may be used, often in conjunction with nonsteroidal anti-inflammatory medications (for arthritis). If the problem is the result of a severely damaged disc, surgery may be needed to relieve the spinal irritation.

A person with MS and back pain should avoid severe spinal manipulation or spinal adjustments (rapid twisting or pushing of the spinal column), because they may irritate the spinal cord, increasing the neurologic problems.

It is critical that a correct diagnosis of the cause of any type of pain be made to ensure that it is properly treated. Diagnostic studies

> *A person with MS and back pain should avoid severe spinal manipulation or spinal adjustments (rapid twisting or pushing of the spinal column).*

that include MRI and computed tomographic (CT) scanning may be needed to pinpoint the cause of the pain.

Other types of musculoskeletal problems of an orthopedic nature are commonly seen in MS. Ligament damage may result if there is too much knee hyperextension during walking. The knee may swell and may be very painful. Many orthopedic specialists are unfamiliar with MS and do not understand why this related problem occurs. As a result, they may recommend exercises such as "quad sets" to increase the strength of the weak leg. Unfortunately, if strength could be put back into the leg, the problem would not have happened in the first place! Exercising the leg with orthopedic exercises actually produces fatigue and increases weakness. Thus, the exercise program fails. A more appropriate approach is to take the load off the leg with an assistive device such as a cane or a crutch. A knee brace may be necessary and helpful to prevent hyperextension.

There has been an explosion of pain management centers. It must be emphasized that simply taking strong pain medication rarely provides for a long-term solution in these difficult situations.

C h a p t e r
17

DIZZINESS AND VERTIGO

The term *vertigo* refers to the sensation of spinning, which, when severe, may be accompanied by nausea and vomiting. There are many causes of vertigo. In MS the problem usually results from an irritation of the brain stem structures that help to maintain balance by coordinating the eyes, arms, and legs. The inner ears also play a major role in balance, and disturbances in the conduction of input to the brain from the inner ear may be very distressing. Dizziness and the sensation of lightheadedness are less severe than vertigo, but nonetheless they cause discomfort. Obviously, other diseases that involve these structures produce similar symptoms, and it should not be assumed that they are necessarily caused by MS.

Antihistamines, including diphenhydramine (Benadryl®), meclizine (Antivert®), and dimenhydrinate (Dramamine®), frequently provide relief when vertigo or sensations of dizziness are relatively mild. Niacin (a component of vitamin B complex) occasionally is used to dilate blood vessels in the hope that this will reduce the problem.

Benzodiazepines, the class of medications that includes diazepam (Valium®), clonazepam (Klonopin®), and oxazepam (Serax®), directly suppress the structures of the inner ear that stimulate dizziness. They are potent antidizziness treatments, but they must be used judiciously. These medications, individually or occasionally in combination, provide sufficient relief to allow the person affected by dizziness to continue functioning reasonably well.

The physical therapy of vertigo has made significant improvements in the past several years. Comprehensive "dizzy" or "vertigo" clinics have become more available and often have special equipment to test and treat dizzy conditions. A physical therapist may teach effective exercises if dizziness is made worse by positional changes. The therapist determines which positions of the head make the dizziness worse. Therapy consists of holding the head in those positions for as long as is tolerated. If this is done successfully, tolerance develops and comfort results. Often, while doing the exercises initially, there is a stimulation and worsening of the dizziness which over time improves. Thus, patience is necessary.

Dizziness frequently accompanies an attack of influenza. When flu and its accompanying fever and muscle aches occur, the symptoms are managed with aspirin or other medication, and the dizziness often disappears as the flu symptoms ease.

If vertigo is severe and vomiting prevents the use of oral medications, intravenous fluids are administered in combination with high doses of cortisone to decrease inflammation in the region that produces these symptoms, the brain stem area at the base of the brain.

Chapter
18

NUMBNESS, COLD FEET, AND SWOLLEN ANKLES

This group of symptoms commonly occur with MS, but they can be managed easily and are not major problems with the disease.

NUMBNESS AND TINGLING

Numbness and tingling are among the most common complaints in MS. They usually are an annoyance rather than a truly disabling symptom. They occur when the nerves that transmit sensation do not conduct information properly, so that one is unable to feel sensation from that area.

Little can be done to treat numbness and, because it usually is a harmless symptom, there is no real need to do so. In some cases steroids may improve sensation by decreasing inflammation, but their use is reserved for instances of real need. Gabapentin (Neurontin®) and/or amitriptyline (Elavil®) may be administered with an occasional decrease in feelings of numbness.

Focusing on numbness may magnify the problem and make it especially bothersome. The best approach is to realize that it is only an annoyance and does not imply a worsening of the disease. A more aggressive approach with cortisone therapy may be considered if the numbness involves the hands, impairing fine movements, or the genitalia, making sexual relations difficult. Unfortunately, no medication specifically treats numbness. If the numbness gets in the way of function, a course of corticosteroids may be necessary.

COLD FEET

The complaint of cold feet is common in MS, even in the milder forms of the disease. The maintenance of skin temperature is an "involuntary" process under the control of that portion of the nervous system referred to as "autonomic," which controls functions such as heart rate, sweating, and pupil dilation. Short-circuiting in the interconnections that control the diameter of blood vessels and those nerves that sense temperature appears to be responsible for the perception of cold feet.

This symptom may be annoying, but it usually is innocuous. There is nothing wrong with the blood vessels themselves in the legs or feet, and there is nothing dangerous in the slight drop in temperature that produces this sensation. It should be emphasized that cold feet do not signify a general circulatory problem. Most people who have this symptom are young and have normal blood vessels. Although they are not protected from vascular disease by MS, they are no more likely to have it than are others of a similar age. Nonetheless, if the problem is severe it should be checked out by a physician. The nerves that work to keep the feet warm may be damaged, and surgical intervention may help you regain control over those nerves. This is unusual but can be of value in those situations.

The best way to manage the problem of cold feet is with warm socks, an electric blanket, and similar local treatments. Occasionally, niacin or medications that dilate blood vessels may be used to alleviate this symptom when it is particularly annoying.

SWOLLEN ANKLES

Swollen ankles result from an accumulation of *lymphatic fluid*, which helps carry nutrients and other substances to and from the organs of the body. This accumulation most often results from reduced activity of the muscles of the leg, which under normal circumstances help keep the fluid moving in the *lymphatic channels* and propel it upward toward the body cavity. When the fluid leaks out of its channels, gravity causes it to pool in the ankles and feet. This problem is common to many diseases in which the use of the legs is reduced. Unless the swelling is extreme, it usually is painless.

"Water pills" (diuretics) usually fail to reduce this type of swelling because they cannot move the fluid upward. If swelling is reduced, the fluid usually returns very soon, even if the medication is continued. Effective treatment is relatively simple and consists of keeping the feet sufficiently elevated so that gravity can begin to move the fluid toward the trunk. This means placing the feet higher than the hips for periods of time during the day and throughout the night. Support stockings may also be of assistance by helping to keep the fluid within its normal channels; these must be fitted properly to avoid pinching the muscles of the leg.

There are also special stockings that are worn at night during sleep and actually pump the fluid back into the system by massaging the muscles of the legs. These are very effective but are expensive and should be reserved for special situations.

Despite the continued leakage of fluid, swollen ankles are essentially a nuisance, requiring looser shoes and so on, rather than a sign of a major problem. Swelling may be more noticeable in summer months because blood vessels and lymph channels dilate (swell) more when the temperature is higher. Sometimes the swelling is severe and does not go away and makes it hard to wear shoes and be comfortable. Specially trained physical therapists who are "lymphedema" specialists can be miraculous at getting the fluid mobilized.

Occasionally, extra fluid may accumulate in the body and pool in the ankles because the heart does not function properly. If a cardiac problem exists, swelling may be accompanied by shortness of breath, coughing, and a general feeling of being unwell. If swelling occurs rapidly, especially in one leg, and is accompanied by redness and pain, it is extremely important to rule out the possibility of *thrombophlebitis* (inflammation of the veins), which may lead to blood clots. This may require special testing. It is therefore important that a physician assess the cause of ankle swelling and determine proper treatment.

C h a p t e r
19

COGNITIVE DIFFICULTIES

Memory, planning, foresight, and judgment are part of what makes us human. This is what we call cognition. The transmission of nerve impulses from the front of the brain to the back, from side to side, and back and forth are what enable memory and communication. This transmission requires highly myelinated fiber tracts working at top efficiency. It should come as no surprise that impairment happens all too often in MS. It is estimated that 50% to 55% of people with MS will have some problem with cognition. About 10% to 15% have significant problems that can lead to decreased job performance and altered social skills. Because this is often a transmission problem, there may be times when it all works well and others when it falls apart. These bad times are worse with heat, stress, and fatigue. The problem is very different from that seen in Alzheimer's disease, which involves across-the-board memory loss. In MS the loss can be very spotty.

Occasionally a person experiences such severe cognitive difficulties that the condition is called "cerebral MS." In cerebral MS the person often has no insight that he or she is experiencing a problem, which makes it more difficult to help.

Prevention is key. We cannot get back what is lost; thus, if there is any indication of cognitive issues, being on a disease-modifying treatment is essential. Cognitive issues are bad prognostic indicators and their presence is enough to warrant aggressive disease-modifying treatments (DMTs).

A key to treatment at this time is *compensation*. It is impossible to get the nerves to start working after they have been damaged. Testing needs to be done to determine one's strengths and weaknesses in order to build on the strengths. The testing can be extensively done by neuropsychologists or less aggressively by speech pathologists or occupational therapists.

It is important to treat aggressively any depression that may complicate the situation, to review all medication taken for MS and other conditions, and to assess the possible effects of each on cognition.

The brain of an adult was once thought to lack what is termed *plasticity*—the ability to switch function to another brain area to allow for restoration of function normally controlled by a damaged area. We now believe that the brain has a greater degree of plasticity than was once thought. How to stimulate this is a great challenge that is being worked on diligently.

A number of compensatory techniques are used to work with the cognitive problems of MS. First, those problems need to be found and their extent measured. This is done through testing, either by a speech pathologist or more formally by a neuropsychologist. Remember that nobody's memory is perfect. Stress, anxiety, and fatigue all decrease cognition, especially memory. Poor concentration may add to the problem. Depression must be treated. A person with MS often does not recognize his or her depression but may respond to medication and therapy. Psychologic tests may be necessary to make the diagnosis of depression.

The following strategies have been found to be helpful in managing cognitive problems:

- Make lists—shopping lists, lists of things to do, and so forth.
- Use a calendar for appointments and reminders of special days.

- Establish a memory notebook to log daily events, reminders, and messages from family and friends.
- Use a tape recorder or voice recorder apps on your mobile phone or computer to help remember information or make up lists.
- Organize your environment so that things remain in familiar places.
- Carry on conversations in quiet places to minimize environmental distractions.
- Ask people to keep directions simple.
- Repeat information and write down important points.
- Establish good eye contact during any discussion.

Cognitive problems may be minimized if a person with such a problem can be made aware that it exists and is willing to change his or her mode of operation by using compensatory techniques. Part of the difficulty is creating this awareness without creating antagonism. This is the age of computers, and both electronic and nonelectronic organizers may be especially helpful in organizing your life.

Cognitive rehabilitation has not been well established for MS as yet, but the beginnings are taking shape. Although cognitive rehabilitation can teach people some ways to compensate, in general it has not become a practical way to counteract the losses of brain demyelination. The best strategy is to prevent the damage from occurring with aggressive earlier treatment with immune modulation.

It would certainly be nice if a medication were available that would decrease cognitive deficits. A number of these have been introduced for Alzheimer's management. However, MS is not Alzheimer's, and these medications appear to have only minor positive effects in MS. Nonetheless, they are fairly easy to take and may be worth a trial. These include donepezil HCl (Aricept®) and memantine (Namenda®). A trial should last a few months, after which all involved need to assess the cost versus benefit of continuing.

It has become quite clear that despite the fact that the brain is not a muscle, if you do not use it, you will lose it. With cognitive problems, people tend to withdraw from society and stop going to movies, to restaurants, to worship services, and so on. As their social contacts diminish, so does brain stimulation. Thus staying active remains an important therapeutic strategy.

P a r t

III

Your Total Health

Chapter

20

DIET AND NUTRITION

No one with multiple sclerosis (MS) can manage at a high level of function without a sound diet and good nutrition. In the many decades of modern MS management, numerous different diets and nutritional supplements have been recommended to those suffering from MS. Some of these are actually opposites in terms of their recommendations, and all have testimonials indicating success. What remains clear is that, at our present state of knowledge, no nutritional treatment available will make much long-term difference in the course of MS.

Most nutritional treatments are benign, but sometimes a fringe-type diet will advocate a nonhealthy regimen. This is especially true when megadoses of any supplement are given. The cost of these forms of treatment may make a safe but noneffective treatment a major economic threat to family survival.

Living a healthy lifestyle and eating sensibly is not difficult but may take some attention to detail. It is very easy to gain weight, especially if exercise has been limited by disability. The body's metabolism decreases, and weight can increase rapidly. Thus, limiting the intake of high-calorie foods, especially sugared drinks, is essential.

Understanding basic concepts of nutrition is helpful. There are six components to the biologic process of life: proteins, carbohydrates, fats, vitamins, minerals, and water.

Amino acids have been called the "building blocks of life" and are put together in various combinations to form proteins. They are involved in many of the chemical and hormonal reactions that go on in the body. They can repair tissue and are involved in growth and development. It takes more energy to metabolize protein than other nutrients. Thus, to decrease caloric intake and maintain weight, many have advocated increasing protein intake at the expense of other nutrients.

Fats are a major source of energy for the body. One gram of fat provides nine calories of energy—more than twice as much as proteins or carbohydrates. Fats help in the absorption of nutrients and provide subcutaneous insulation for the body. Saturated fats from animals are solid at room temperature (e.g., butter and lard). Unsaturated fats include corn and olive oil, which are liquid at room temperature and are derived from plants. Fat intake should be heavier on the unsaturated fat side because saturated fats increase cholesterol levels and thus the risk for heart disease.

Carbohydrates are necessary for muscles to metabolize fat for energy. Carbohydrates are formed from sugar molecules that link together and make the complex carbohydrates called starch found in many vegetables. Blood sugar is controlled by the breakdown of carbohydrates and the release of sugar.

Vitamins are necessary for the metabolic process that results in the breakdown of carbohydrate and fat to make energy. They are classified as fat soluble (vitamins A, D, E, and K) and water soluble (vitamins B, vitamin C). Fat-soluble vitamins are absorbed from the GI tract in the presence of fat and can be stored in fat tissue. It is possible to ingest toxic doses of the fat-soluble vitamins by taking megadoses of them. Water-soluble vitamins usually are excreted by the kidneys and, if overdosed, rarely cause problems, although high doses of vitamin C can lead to gastric distress and occasionally kidney/bladder stones.

More than 20 different minerals are essential for the body to function optimally. These include calcium, phosphorus, iodine, magnesium, and zinc. They strengthen bones and teeth and make the chemistry of the body more efficient.

There are many who advocate large doses and unusual combinations of vitamins and minerals for all that ails humans. While no vitamin can be called "the MS vitamin," vitamin D is becoming close to that. As mentioned in Chapter 1, recent studies have found a correlation between vitamin D deficiency and MS. This is a very fertile area of research now and into the future. In the interval the question remains as to whether those at risk in areas away from the equator, where reduced sunlight causes lower natural levels of vitamin D, or those with MS should be on high doses of vitamin D. No one has the absolutely correct answer but it appears that fairly high doses of vitamin D are well tolerated and not expensive. Many MS professionals recommend doses around 4000 to 5000 IU per day.

Sixty percent to seventy percent of the body is composed of water. It is essential to transport nutrients, remove waste, and regulate temperature. Many "experts" have advocated drinking eight glasses of water a day, but there is no magic number. Drinking enough to satisfy thirst and prevent dehydration, along with preventing constipation, is necessary and may differ from person to person.

Many diets have been advocated for persons with MS, including contradictory ones (e.g., low-carbohydrate versus high-carbohydrate). What is important is to make sure that your diet is well balanced and allows for a good and happy quality of life. The Internet has emphasized some clearly ridiculous ideas of what may make MS worse. Aspartame clearly has nothing to do with MS, but may irritate the bladder wall, causing increased frequency of urination. Caffeine does a similar number on the bladder. Mercury intoxication is a bad thing, but does not look like MS and has nothing to do with amalgams in the mouth used for fillings. One can understand this lack of association simply by looking at MS before and after these substances were introduced to humans and noting that nothing changed before or after.

In the previous editions of this book, Dr. Daniel Kosich expressed some dietary guidelines, which remain of import and are therefore reproduced here:

1. Eat a wide variety of foods.
   - Choose daily from each of the five basic food groups according to servings recommended. (see Figure 20.1)
   - Emphasize adequate amounts of foods high in complex carbohydrates: whole grains and a wide variety of vegetables and fruits each day.

2. Avoid too much dietary fat (especially saturated) and cholesterol.
   - Read food labels.
   - Eat low-fat dairy foods.
   - Eat lean cuts of meat such as flank steak, lean round steak, ocean fish (except smelt), and skinless poultry. Limit meat consumption to three to four ounces per day.
   - Limit the amount of fat added to foods (butter, oils, dressings, and spreads).
   - Bake, broil, and boil instead of frying.

3. Reduce simple sugar intake (table sugar, molasses, honey, corn syrup, refined and processed foods, and so on).
   - Drink less canned soda and sweetened beverages.
   - DRINK MORE WATER!
   - Use seasonings to replace sugar in recipes: e.g., vanilla extract, cinnamon, allspice, cardamom, nutmeg, mint, mace, clove, and ginger.

4. Avoid too much sodium.
   - Many foods provide sodium. Add less than one-half teaspoon of salt per day to your food. Eat a variety of vegetables and whole grains.
   - Use these foods to add a "salty" flavor to recipes: onion, garlic, parsley, celery, cayenne, chili powder, rosemary, sage, tarragon, oregano, and basil.

5. If you drink alcohol, do so in moderation (no more than one to two ounces per day).

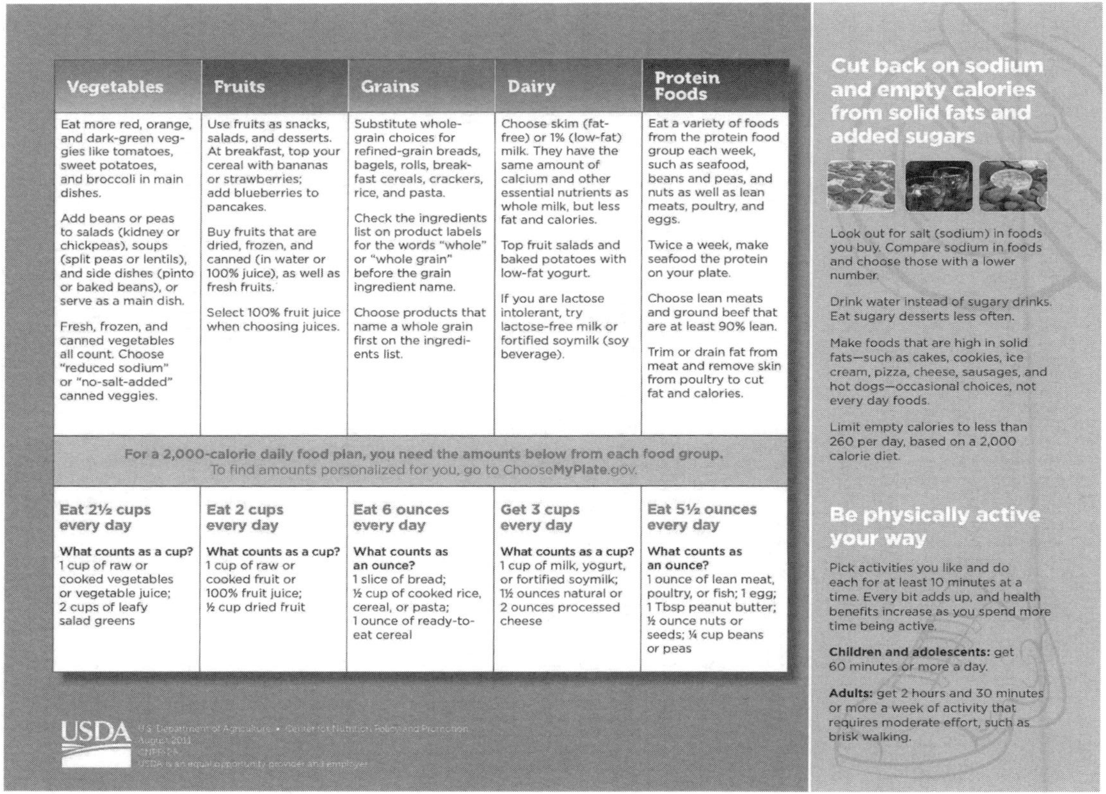

FIGURE 20.1 USDA five food groups. Adapted from the USDA Center for Nutrition Policy and Promotion's ChooseMyPlate.gov website.

WEIGHT CONTROL

A common concern of everyone, including those who have MS, is how to achieve and maintain a healthy body weight. In addition to good nutrition, activity is crucial.

Often, especially when the capability to exercise is limited, the choice is made to help regulate body weight by not eating very much. This may be risky because eating enough of the right kinds of foods is as important as exercise in overall weight management. Most often, very low-calorie diets do not lead to effective weight control in the long run, but may actually make the body store more fat.

Low-Calorie Dieting

1. The body quickly begins to decrease its basic calorie expenditure (the basal metabolic rate) to conserve energy. Thus, fewer calories are burned, not more.
2. The body does not function properly without enough carbohydrate, and it begins to convert muscle protein to carbohydrate so that it can continue to make energy. Losing muscle tissue is not desirable. Of a 10-pound weight loss in two weeks on a low-carbohydrate diet, only approximately two to three pounds are fat because approximately five pounds are water and two to three pounds are lost from muscle.
3. While all this is going on, the body is increasing its ability to store fat when it gets enough calories sometime in the future. This is a basic survival mechanism for times of inadequate food intake, but it is not desirable when the goal is weight loss or weight maintenance.

It certainly is possible to lose weight on a low-calorie diet. However, the period of rapid weight loss typically lasts only about a week or two, and then it stops. During that period the body "readjusts" its metabolism to survive on fewer calories. When a more normal caloric intake resumes, the body takes advantage of its increased "fat-storing" ability to increase its energy reserves in stored body fat. The weight lost as water and muscle is not replaced as water and muscle; it is replaced as fat. Over time, even though total weight may not actually change significantly, the percent of body fat may increase dramatically. This clearly is not the desired goal.

Because of the associated risks and poor long-term success rate, low-calorie diets should only be attempted under the supervision of a physician. Keep in mind that in the long run, success most likely will be achieved by eating enough of the right kinds of foods and by being as active as possible within the limits of your individual situation.

> *Because of the associated risks and poor long-term success rate, low-calorie diets should only be attempted under the supervision of a physician.*

Reading Nutrition Labels

One of the easiest ways to keep track of the amount of fat is to read nutrition labels to determine the percentage of calories in a food item provided by fat.

To quickly read the label on a prepared food item, just remember that each gram of fat provides nine calories.

$$1 \text{ gram of fat} = 9 \text{ calories}$$

Take the following label as an example:

Nutritional information per serving (2 tbsp)
Calories per serving = 210
Carbohydrate = 5 grams
Protein = 10 grams
Fat = 18 grams

To find the number of calories supplied by fat:

1. Multiply the grams of fat by 9:

$$18 \times 9 = 162 \text{ calories}$$

Divide the number of calories from fat by the total calories to determine the percent of calories from fat:

$$162/210 = 77\%$$

Therefore, this food item (peanut butter) is approximately 75% fat calories. Does that mean it is a "bad" food? No, it simply suggests that it should be eaten in moderation.

Remember that of all the food eaten each day, approximately 20% to 25% of the calories should be from fat. Any one food item (such as peanut butter) that is high in fat should be eaten only in small quantities.

A sensible nutritional lifestyle is simply a question of balancing the appropriate number of servings from USDA's MyPlate. Peanut butter, because of its high fat content, would not appear on the plate and is considered an occasional choice. Put it on two slices of whole grain bread (from the grains portion of the plate) to make a nutritious sandwich. Add a carrot, an apple, and a glass of skim milk and you have a great lunch!

Some examples of fat contents of foods are shown in Table 20.1.

CUTTING FAT CALORIES

Because reducing the amount of dietary fat is important for both health and weight control, here are some reinforcements and specific suggestions on ways to reduce the amount of dietary fat:

- Decrease or omit butter, margarine, spreads, mayonnaise, and salad dressings. Remember that each gram of fat eliminated also eliminates nine calories. Using one teaspoon of dressing instead of one tablespoon reduces the fat calories by 67 percent!
- Change the way foods are prepared. Deep-frying greatly increases the fat content of many foods. Learn to bake, broil, boil, and microwave, and use nonstick cooking pans.

TABLE 20.1   Examples of Food Labels

Food Item	Quantity	Calories	Fat (g)	% Fat
Milk (4%)	1 cup	150	9	54
Milk (2%)	1 cup	120	5	38
Milk (skim)	1 cup	90	1	10
Cottage cheese (whole milk)	1/2 cup	120	5	38
Cottage cheese (1% milk)	1/2 cup	90	1	10
Yogurt, plain (whole milk)	1 cup	160	7	31
Yogurt, plain (1% milk)	8 oz	140	3	15
Granola bar (sugars are 7 out of 13 ingredients!)	1	140	7	35
Candy bar	1	270	13	43
Butter	1 tbsp	100	9	99
Margarine	1 tbsp	100	10	56

- Decrease the amount of meat you consume. Most meats, especially red meats, contain more fat calories than protein calories. For that reason it is important to select fish, poultry, and lean cuts of beef, such as rump, round, and flank.
- Be aware that many dairy products are high in fat. For instance, whole milk (labeled as 4% milk fat) actually contains approximately 50% fat calories because of the caloric density of fat. Cheeses made with whole milk often have 75% or more of their calories from fat. Therefore, it is important to select from low-fat dairy products, such as skim milk and 1% milk and yogurt and cheeses made with low-fat milk. If you have lactose intolerance, ask your doctor if taking milk products with Lactaid® might allow the nutritional benefits of dairy foods.

Any food may be eaten in moderation. Appreciate it for what it is, enjoy it, and blend it into a sensible nutritional lifestyle.

Perhaps the most important consideration is that you decide what kinds of foods you eat. It is not easy to change habits, and tastes take a long time to change. Be patient; good eating is in everyone's best interest.

The key is moderation. Any food may be eaten in moderation. Appreciate it for what it is, enjoy it, and blend it into a sensible nutritional lifestyle.

WEIGHT GAIN

Weight gain may be a problem in MS if your activity level drops but your caloric intake remains constant. Very few people who are overweight do not know it; there is little point to making continuous comments about it to an overweight individual. No data indicate that weight gain causes or is associated with weakness, but it is not good for your overall health and is unattractive to many people. It may make general movement more difficult than necessary especially aided transfers.

People who are overweight usually would like to be thinner, but they often can do very little to change the situation. Decreasing caloric intake only works to a certain extent for people with limited mobility and a decreased level of activity. Understanding that one sometimes has to deal with a situation the way it is and not fret over what cannot be done makes for a better quality of life.

A number of exercises can be done from chairs or beds to keep limber and increase muscle tone. It takes real ambition to stick to an exercise program, but it is quite important. People who use a wheelchair often appear to have weight gain in the abdomen, but this is an unavoidable result of not being able to do enough repetitions of stomach-firming exercises.

The same basic dietary guidelines that apply to others also apply to people with MS.

The same basic dietary guidelines that apply to others also apply to people with MS. Appetite suppressants have little long-term effect. You must strive for a balance between exercise, calories, and fatigue. This starts with eating smaller meals. Many people find that eating small but frequent meals results in both lower overall caloric intake and greater satisfaction.

Chapter

21

EXERCISE

Sometimes people with MS are told to rest and not overdo, and the fear of fatigue may become almost unbearable. There is no real basis for this fear. *People with MS are not fragile!* Good clinical studies have shown that proper exercise increases fitness and reduces fatigue.

The principles of exercise for those with MS have changed as more knowledge has accumulated. Jimmie Heuga, a former Olympic skier, was influential in this area. Founder of the The Jimmie Heuga Center for Multiple Sclerosis, now called Can Do MS, Heuga showed that modern physical fitness training techniques and appropriate aerobic exercise could benefit those with MS.

The "no pain, no gain" philosophy applies only to certain situations. Typically the process is slow and begins with a carefully developed exercise prescription. Like medication, it should be prescribed by a professional, usually a physical therapist or a physician who knows how to develop exercises for a specific individual.

The exercise prescription should have four elements:

1. The *type* of exercise (aerobic, strengthening, balance, coordination, stretching, and so on)
2. The *duration* of exercise (how long you should exercise)
3. The *frequency* of exercise (how often you should exercise)
4. The *intensity* of exercise (how hard you should exercise)

The role of exercise in MS has become somewhat controversial, partly because the meaning of the term exercise is misunderstood. To many people, *exercise* is defined as stressing their bodies to the point of pain, expressed by the phrase "no pain, no gain." But it has become quite clear that if a person with MS exercises to the point of pain, fatigue will set in and weakness will increase.

> *The role of exercise in MS has become somewhat controversial, partly because the meaning of the term exercise is misunderstood.*

Rigorous exercise also increases the core body temperature (as opposed to superficial skin temperature). The myelin coating that normally surrounds nerves protects them from the effects of this rise in temperature. Because of the loss of myelin in MS, a rise in core body temperature increases the amount of short-circuiting in the CNS, worsening existing symptoms and sometimes producing new ones. This is why exercise originally fell into bad repute with those who are knowledgeable about MS.

Our understanding of what is "good" exercise for people with MS and how they should train has increased considerably in the past few years as the concept of overall "fitness" has developed. Fitness is a holistic concept that implies general overall health, the goal of which is improved function of the heart, lungs, muscles, and

> *It is important to tailor an exercise program for each individual rather than have a set program for everyone who has the disease.*

other organs. It is attained by proper diet, by not smoking, and by exercising appropriately.

Two major concepts underlie the term *appropriate* exercise. First, because of the wide variability of the disease, what is good exercise for one person may not be good exercise for another. It is important to tailor an exercise program for each individual rather than have a set program for everyone who has the disease. The second concept is that there are many kinds of exercise—exercise does not mean only running, jumping, or similar aerobic activities.

More work is required to move stiff muscles, resulting in early fatigue and increased weakness. Exercises that increase mobility through stretching and maintaining range of motion are discussed in Chapter 5, and a series of basic exercises is given in Appendix A. These exercises play an important part in combating weakness by reducing the stiffness that so commonly is present in MS.

Balance exercises are discussed in Chapter 7. These exercises are very different from those that are used to reduce spasticity. If balance is a problem, muscles must use more energy to maintain an upright stance, and anything that increases balance will therefore reduce weakness.

Relaxation exercises are discussed in Chapter 23. A person who is under stress will experience an increase in weakness. For this reason, techniques for learning how to relax should be part of any overall program designed to reduce weakness and fatigue.

Aerobic exercises are what most people think of as "real" exercise. They may involve using a bicycle, rowing machine, or treadmill, brisk walking or running, or a brisk self-wheel in a wheelchair. It is important to understand that the word *aerobic* implies that the body is taking in enough oxygen to meet its needs in the exercise program. This is compared with the anaerobic state that occurs when a person exercises too aggressively and starves the body of oxygen. *Endurance increases slowly but surely under aerobic conditions.*

Specifically, you should be able to speak a sentence out loud during any aerobic exercise (except perhaps swimming). Enough air should be available to permit clear and somewhat effortless speaking. If you cannot speak in this fashion, it is likely that the type or extent of the exercise is anaerobic and harmful.

The proper exercise prescription takes into account that no exercise should cause pain. "No pain, no gain" is absolutely the wrong approach to exercise for the person with MS. The proper exercise prescription is a balanced one that includes many different types of exercises with the goal of improving overall condition. With such an improvement, a parallel gain in strength is to be expected.

> *"No pain, no gain" is absolutely the wrong approach to exercise for the person with MS.*

Chapter

22

SEXUALITY

Sexuality is a complex part of life, one that is difficult to define or measure because its expression is special and private for each individual. It has its roots in being human and adds a richness and pleasure to life that goes far beyond the sexual act. Although our society has recently become more open about sex and sexuality, many myths and negative attitudes still exist concerning the sexuality of those who have a chronic illness such as MS. Many people think that a diagnosis of MS means that their sexual life has ended, that it somehow is wrong or "inappropriate" to continue having sexual needs or to seek information about maintaining a satisfying sexual life.

Sexuality does and should continue to be an important part of life for people with MS. Sexuality affects your basic feelings of self-esteem and your views of yourself as masculine or feminine. It provides pleasure and relaxation, and it is an important aspect of relationships with a spouse or significant other because sharing a sexual life strengthens the attachment between partners.

A chronic illness such as MS may have a tremendous impact on sexuality. Sexual functioning—the actual physiology and mechanics of sex—may be affected by physical changes resulting from illness-related neurologic changes or by the presence of symptoms such as spasticity, bowel and bladder problems, pain, and fatigue.

The psychological feelings associated with coping with an illness such as MS, including anxiety and depression, also may interfere with sexual expression and desire. Additionally, the partner of an individual who is coping with illness may experience a similar range of feelings, which may interfere with his or her sexual ability and interest. Although there may be changes in sexuality in reaction to MS, sexual needs neither disappear nor become inappropriate. This chapter discusses both possible changes in sexuality that may occur as the result of MS and strategies to obtain information and maintain a positive sense of sexuality in the presence of the disease.

THE SEXUAL RESPONSE

The sexual response depends on a complicated series of reflexes that involve the neuromuscular transmissions stimulated by a wide variety of visual, tactile (touch), olfactory (smell), and emotional sensations. Sexual excitement and response begin in the brain. Electrical signals are transmitted from the brain areas involved via the spinal cord to the sexual organs or genitals, through nerves that exit near the base of the spinal cord. The pathways between the brain and the genitals are long and complex, and demyelination may "short-circuit" them.

Impulses leave the CNS from the sacral spinal cord via the autonomic nervous system, which controls bodily functions that are considered "automatic." For example, this system controls the arousal that men and women experience without external stimulation, such as that which occurs during sleep. There are two divisions to the autonomic nervous system, the *parasympathetic* and the *sympathetic*. The parasympathetic section controls the erectile response. Erections in men may be stimulated by visual stimuli. Obviously, for a visual stimulus to cause an erection, there must be an intact pathway from the brain down the spinal cord to the sexual organs. Demyelination may interfere with the connections from the "brain erection center" to the target organ, the penis.

There is clear evidence of a spinal center for erection as well as the brain center. As a result, reflex erections still may occur, but even when desired, willed erections may become impossible. Stimulation of the penis by masturbation or as part of sexual foreplay may allow an erection to occur if the pathway from the penis to the spinal cord and within the spinal cord back to the penis remains intact. This stimulation may require greater intensity if there is numbness or if sensation to the stimulus is decreased. Finally, erections may occur during sleep that may or may not be controlled by these centers.

The normal male sexual response has three phases: desire, lubrication/swelling (excitement, plateau phases), and orgasm. The first response to sexual stimulation is erection, which is accompanied by increases in muscle tension, heart rate, blood pressure, and respiration. This then "plateaus" with advanced lubrication and swelling and is followed by a series of contractions by which the sympathetic nervous system allows for ejaculation (emission). Finally, the body returns to its resting state during the resolution stage.

The penis has soft, spongy tissue that easily expands when it is filled with blood. The tip of the penis, the bulb, is very sensitive to stimulation and sends messages to the various centers if it is appropriately stimulated. These centers allow the parasympathetic system to be stimulated, causing blood to be trapped within the spongy tissue of the penis to produce an erection. Ejaculation, the expulsion of liquid (semen) from the penis, is handled by the sympathetic division. When the stimulus ends or ejaculation occurs, the blood flows out of the penis and the erection disappears.

The external female genitalia, or vulva, consists of the labia majora (large outer lips of the vagina), the labia minora (smaller inner lips), the clitoris, and the vestibule. Like the male penis, the clitoris contains spongy tissue and a significant number of blood vessels. Bartholin glands, which produce a lubrication fluid, lie adjacent to the vagina.

As in men, the phases of normal female sexual response include desire, lubrication/swelling (excitement and plateau phase), and orgasm. The factors involved in the desire phase are not well understood but clearly may be affected by MS. Increased sexual excitement is accompanied by muscle tension, increased blood flow to the clitoris, and the beginning of vaginal lubrication, which then plateaus with increased lubrication and swelling. Orgasm consists of rhythmic contractions of the muscles around the vagina and uterus.

SEXUAL PROBLEMS IN MULTIPLE SCLEROSIS

Given the complexity of the sexual response in terms of the neuro-muscular transmissions involved, it is no surprise that sexual difficulties often are encountered in MS. Such difficulties frequently are clearly physical, although a psychological component may be involved in many or most instances of difficulty.

More than 90% of all men with MS and more than 70% of all women with MS report some change in their sexual life after the onset of the disease. Men most often report impaired genital sensation, decreased sexual drive, inability or difficulty in achieving and maintaining an erection, and delayed ejaculation or decreased force of ejaculation. Women report impaired genital sensation, diminished orgasmic response, and loss of sexual interest; they also may be bothered by intense itching, diminished vaginal lubrication, weak vaginal muscles, and a reflex pulling together of the legs (adductor spasms).

MANAGING SEXUAL DIFFICULTIES

The diagnosis of MS may alter one's self-image, and it is common to feel sexually unattractive when one is concerned about braces, wheelchairs, and catheters. Perhaps the single most helpful approach to managing sexual difficulties is to focus on becoming comfortable with your body, a goal that requires time and commitment. It is important to identify your positive personal qualities and to put effort into feeling good about yourself by taking care of your body through exercise, diet, dress, and so forth. Feeling good about yourself will help to defeat the myth that you must have a "perfect" body to be sexually attractive.

It cannot be stressed enough that communication is critical to achieving a positive, enjoyable sexual relationship, and feelings must be dealt with openly and honestly. The communication must occur between partners but also with the health care professional. Sometimes this is embarrassing and scary but it needs to take place.

With your partner, it is important to convey information about what feels pleasurable and what does not and to experiment with different sexual positions and creative, alternative ways to give and receive pleasure. Our society emphasizes "normal" or proper ways to obtain sexual gratification, which tends to make sex goal-oriented toward intercourse and orgasm. However, many people find great physical and psychological satisfaction from activities that traditionally have been termed foreplay. One excellent way to decrease or completely eliminate pressures and expectations is to become less goal-oriented by renaming such activities sexplay. Sexual expression may be directed to parts of the body other than the genitals, increasing cuddling, caressing, massage, or other forms of touch, and it may involve experimenting with oral sex, masturbation, a vibrator, or other devices.

Emotional reactions may be an issue for both the person with MS and his or her partner because anxiety, guilt, anger, depression, and denial are the natural consequences of coping with any chronic illness. Again, communication between partners is the key to managing such feelings. Couples should be sensitive to the fact that some painful feelings may not improve or disappear with communication and support. In that case, it may be helpful to seek professional help in response to depression or anxiety that will not go away.

To avoid bowel, bladder, and catheter problems during intercourse, fluids should be reduced approximately two hours before sexual activity and the bladder should be emptied before lovemaking. Be prepared in case an accident occurs despite these precautions, and remember that it is not a catastrophe. If a catheter is used, it may be taped over a man's penis or to a woman's abdomen. A vaginal lubricant such as K-Y jelly should be used whether a woman uses a catheter or not.

Spasticity or leg spasms may be minimized by timing antispasticity medication so that it is maximally effective during sexual activity. Having intercourse in a side position, with the knees bent or using pillows for support, may make a difference and should be tried.

A vibrator may compensate for a loss of deep pressure sense, which is reflected as impaired sensation, numbness, and tingling. A number of different types are available, including hand-held, penis-shaped, and others. They are easily obtained via the Internet. A device called "Eros" has been approved by the FDA for sexual dysfunction in the female. It places gentle suction on the clittoral region while applying a gentle vibration. The judicious use of a frozen bag of peas rubbed gently in the vaginal area has been reported to increase sensation and decrease pain for some people. Lubrication difficulties in women may be managed by vaginal packets of lubricants that open on impact, such as Replens or Astroglide.

Several alternatives are available if a man's erections are insufficient for penetration and intercourse. The use of surgically implanted penile prostheses has decreased dramatically as non-surgical alternatives have become popular. A solid erection may be obtained in most men with injectable prostaglandin, or Caverjet™, which is injected using a small needle approximately 30 minutes before intercourse and almost always creates a strong erection.

An alternative involves the same prostaglandin medication administered into the opening of the penis (urethra) via an applicator. This system, which is called MUSE, is available by prescription. It usually gives an adequate erection with stimulation from one's partner. A rubber band placed at the base of the penis after erection occurs may hold the erection for a longer period of time.

There are many penile vacuum devices, which consist of a tube that is placed over the penis with a rubber band around the top of the tube. A pump removes the air from the tube, creating a vacuum that draws blood into the penis to produce an erection. When the erection is adequate, the rubber band is slid onto the base of the penis and the tube is removed. The erection produced by this method is not as firm as an erection produced by other methods, but it may be adequate for many people.

No medication has been proven to stimulate ejaculation, but the antidepressant trazodone has been reported to be helpful for some people when used at a dose of 5 to 10 mg one hour before intercourse. Testosterone injections and the Eastern drug yohimbine have been used with variable but not encouraging success. Sildenafil (Viagra®), Vardenafil (Levitra®), and tadalafil (Cialis®) often allow for a good erection and have become a major advance in the management of erectile dysfunction. They may be taken by mouth 30 to 60 minutes before intercourse. Absorption is faster if it is crushed and swallowed. It must be understood that foreplay is essential to its working. Cialis has a longer half-life and thus may stay active for one to two days.

Although great strides have been made in diagnosing sexual difficulties and providing alternatives, the key remains good communication between partners and between the person with MS and his or her health care team. By exploring options, requesting information, and seeking appropriate referral, a satisfying sexual life may be maintained while coping with the diagnosis of MS.

Chapter
23

Adapting to Multiple Sclerosis

Adapting to MS begins when the first symptom appears. It usually is vague—mild numbness, some tingling, possibly a feeling of weakness, or occasionally some urgency of urination. The initial impulse is to deny the problem and ignore it. However, if the symptoms persist, fear overcomes denial, often accompanied by self-directed anger. The fear is that of "going crazy," of believing that nothing really is wrong, that it is "all in my head."

Often the opinions of several physicians are sought, including family doctors, internists, and neurologists. Some physicians are vague about the problem, refraining from giving it a name, whereas others may mention MS. Stress and fear build until the tests are completed and the diagnosis is confirmed. This often is followed by a sense of relief that the problem is medical rather than psychological.

However, this relief soon disappears, and anger accompanied by grief surfaces once again. These feelings often are directed somewhat randomly, sometimes toward family, friends, or physicians, as if they were responsible for the disease. A lack of understanding leads to more anger, fear, and resentment, and a "why me?" feeling tends to develop.

Some parallels may be drawn between the process of adjustment to MS and the stages of grief, as described by Elisabeth Kübler-Ross in her book *On Death and Dying*. She observed that people initially deny that death will occur. This is followed by anger, then by a bargaining stage, which in turn evolves into depression, and finally into acceptance. The order may vary, but the process is fairly constant. Family and close friends also go through this adjustment process, and children may follow suit in their own way.

As grieving evolves into depression in the person newly diagnosed with MS, it may be accompanied by loss of sleep, change of appetite, and feelings of despondency. This sequence results from decreased self-esteem; changes in self-image, life plans, goals, and values; and frequently a fear of rejection by family and friends. Resolution of these feelings is hoped for at the end of the cycle, accompanied by the feeling of peace that comes with the understanding that life must go on.

Dr. David Welch shared with me the stages of development in understanding MS he has observed:

1. *Admission.* The individual allows him or herself to admit the reality of MS. This admission is private and involves no one else. Implicit in this admission is that from that moment on all relationships will in some way be altered.
2. *Acknowledgment.* Eventually the fact that one has MS is reluctantly disclosed. Other people need to know if they are to respond properly to the person with MS.
3. *Accommodation.* The disease requires the subordination of some things to the requirements of others.
4. *Adaptation.* The environment needs to be modified to suit the conditions. The world needs to be changed to suit the person with MS, not the reverse.

There are a number of ways to deal with all the adjustments required by MS. The element of stress is constant throughout all phases of the adjustment process. Its effect on the actual demyelination process is unclear, but in all likelihood stress does not increase demyelination. A flare-up of MS symptoms in a person under stress is not a true exacerbation caused by increasing demyelination, despite the fact that stress clearly enhances the symptoms caused by demyelination. The brain has remarkable powers to compensate for the effects of disease, but it often loses this ability when one is under stress. Symptoms that previously were compensated for will then be uncovered. The person with MS therefore will appear to have increased symptoms and problems, which may in turn lead to more stress. It is therefore important that ways of coping with stress be developed.

> *The brain has remarkable powers to compensate for the effects of disease, but it often loses this ability when one is under stress.*

Under normal conditions, stress usually forces one to change and readjust one's outlook. However, the chronic stress that accompanies a disease such as MS may instead result in continued decompensation and maladaptation. This only perpetuates the stress, and the stress–illness relationship becomes quite complicated. Simply put, the stress feeds the illness, and the illness feeds the stress.

All of this results in an angry and despondent person. Anger is what shows on the outside, but depression is the internal mood. The person feels betrayed by his or her own body. The anger alienates others just when their support is most needed. This cycle has led to the perception of an "MS personality." There is no evidence that a specific personality exists in people with MS. Rather, a loss of self-esteem brought on by the perceived loss of physical function leads to mourning these losses, which in turn results in the development of personality traits that may be perceived as very different from those of the "predisease" state.

It is important to understand that MS is actually a disease of the central nervous system, which includes the brain. That means that the MS process by itself will change the biochemistry of the brain. This may result in what appear to be emotional changes, but are really biochemical changes that result in a change in feelings and behavior. Because these are neurochemical, they usually require neurochemical treatment with antidepressants or similar agents. They require some skill on the part of the physician to understand and use the proper medications. They require understanding by the person with MS that a problem exists and that it needs help. All too often the person does not see or feel the difference and the family has to point out how differently he or she is behaving.

Very occasionally, the bulk of the demyelination associated with MS occurs within the brain, and intellect ("smartness") actually decreases. Memory, planning, and foresight diminish, and the personality changes. Initially these changes are subtle, but they increase with time. Emotional lability is the hallmark of this type of disease, with inappropriate episodes of crying and/or laughing. Older memories are lost last in this type of MS, whereas remembering recent events presents the most difficulty. These changes are the result of demyelination rather than psychological causes. Thus, counseling for this problem must be focused on understanding and adjustment. Counseling family and friends can lead to better understanding. Antidepressants may help in controlling some of the emotional lability, whereas tranquilizers sometimes are necessary to control behavior. *It is important to emphasize that this type of MS is rare.*

Most lifestyle stresses caused by MS are helped by appropriate counseling. Many people with MS do not want to recognize the psychological component, and counseling must be subtly offered or it will be strongly refused. Coping skills must be developed on an individual basis; they cannot be learned simply from reading a book. These skills involve learning to deal effectively with stereotypes of the disabled in the community, perceived changes in masculinity or femininity, changes in relationships, changes of roles within the family, changes in employment status, increased dependence on others, and changes in physical condition. Some practical coping techniques include:

- Make a list of conditions required for positive self-esteem, and discipline yourself to create at least some of them.
- Determine a way (small or large) to contribute to society and follow through with your plans.
- Attend appropriate counseling sessions.
- Learn to say no to certain requests in such a way as not to damage your self-esteem.
- Make a list of people who can be relied on for various kinds of support and call on them for assistance when feelings of despair appear.
- Discipline yourself to stay as healthy and as physically fit as possible.
- Create opportunities to get out of the house.
- Take charge of situations rather than allowing them to dictate to you.
- Prioritize projects.

Relaxation Techniques

Although stress usually is viewed as something to be avoided, realistically the key is to learn proper ways to manage unavoidable stress. Some stress is desirable—it energizes us, motivates us, and captivates our interest. The stress that must be managed is the "distress" that may hamper our ability to cope with the events and people in our lives.

Body and mind are linked, and stress affects both our physical and emotional well-being. Stress may produce physical signs such as "knotting" of the stomach, increased spasticity, headaches, tight or sore muscles in the neck, and an increased pulse rate. If left unchecked, more severe symptoms will appear, such as insomnia, fatigue, anxiety, poor concentration, and poor problem-solving abilities.

Relaxation techniques provide a tool with which stress can be controlled, putting you in better overall control of your life and your well-being. *Relaxation takes practice!* To be successful, you must learn to keep a passive attitude and let go of thoughts that drift in and out of your mind. The following steps should be practiced until they become second nature.

> *Although stress usually is viewed as something to be avoided, realistically the key is to learn proper ways to manage unavoidable stress.*

- Begin by finding a quiet place where you will be undisturbed for half an hour or so.
- Sit with your arms, head, and feet supported, or lie down.
- Close your eyes. You may wish to turn on soft music.
- Focus on your breathing. The goal is deep, steady, smooth, and rhythmic breathing.
- Relax your muscles by working systematically through your body. Tell yourself to relax your feet, calf muscles, thighs, buttocks, abdomen, chest, arms, hands, neck, and head. Let your body become heavier and heavier with each breath.
- Now imagine yourself in a pleasant setting. Guide yourself on a fantasy trip to a place you always wanted to see or revisit. Explore this place with all of your senses.
- When you have spent enough time there, leave knowing that you can return at will. Slowly open your eyes and enjoy the calm.

Individual counseling is helpful when you are having difficulty making the necessary adaptations, when you have a lot of anger, when depression becomes an ongoing problem, when self-esteem fails, or when you have difficulty accepting the existence of MS. Group counseling may be helpful when you think that no one understands your problems or if your support system is inadequate.

Having MS and raising children brings about new challenges. They begin with explaining to the kids that MS is unpredictable and variable and that they are not responsible for how the disease runs. They need to know that people do not die from MS and that the average life span is about as long as for those without the disease. Children may have to shoulder increased responsibility within the family, but care must be taken to remember that they are children and need to grow and develop in the best manner possible.

What and/or when to tell your employer about MS is a personal decision that can have many ramifications. It should not but usually does have ramifications associated with the timing of disclosure. Clearly, if job accommodations are desired, a frank discussion is necessary. However, if there is no accommodation wanted and if job performance is not impaired, it might be better to keep one's personal health, in general, personal. When interviewing, the situation must be sized up. Your physician may be able to give advice for specific circumstances, but in the end it will be up to each individual to find the right time and give accurate information so as not to make a difficult situation worse.

The person with MS need not go through life waiting for "the other shoe to drop." By understanding some of the psychological changes that accompany chronic disease, you may take an active role to achieve a healthy mental state. The physically challenged must also win the "mental/emotional" challenge. There is no simple way to do this, but it is clear that if one surrenders, one loses!

Chapter

24

Aging with Multiple Sclerosis

While there are exceptions, people die with MS, not from MS. The average life expectancy for all with MS (severe and not severe) is only a few years less than those without the disease. Therefore, aging with a neurological disease becomes an issue over time. It may be a bit controversial but, for the most part, MS tends to slow down in terms of progression as people get into their 60s. This is true for most autoimmune diseases as the immune system appears to poop out to some degree. There are many exceptions to the rule but many who have various amounts of disability will find the progression to be much slower as they age. However, they do continue to age. It can be stated that there is not much difference between those who are 40 and 50 without MS. There is not much difference between 50 and 60 years of age. But there is a difference between 60 and 70 years of age and a significant difference for most between 70 and 80.

Walking may become more difficult, not because of MS progression, but because the aging nervous system simply does not have the reserve it should have and, as it ages, problems are magnified. The aging bladder has been written about for decades and having MS does not protect one from those issues. Hormonal changes surrounding menopause are unpredictable but often there are issues that need some compensation. Osteoporosis is a problem for chronic disease in general and with aging may become more problematic. Cognitive issues may become magnified.

All of these naturally occurring events have some management strategies that are not unique to MS. The answer to disability continues to be mobility and that becomes truer with aging. Having appropriate medical and physical/occupational therapy follow-up becomes essential with the aging nervous system.

It truly is wonderful that the opportunity to age with MS is here and there are things to be done to improve all quality of life, no matter what the age.

Part

IV

APPENDICES

Appendix
A

GLOSSARY

Abductor muscle—A muscle used to pull a body part away from the midline of the body (e.g., the abductor leg muscles are used to spread the legs).

ACTH—Adrenocorticotropic hormone; a hormone produced by the pituitary gland that stimulates the adrenal glands to produce cortisone.

Adductor muscle—A muscle that pulls inward toward the midline of the body (e.g., the adductor leg muscles are used to pull the legs together).

Affective disorder—A disturbance of mood in an individual, such as depression.

Amino acids—Compounds composed of carbon, nitrogen, and an acid; the building blocks of proteins.

Amyotrophic lateral sclerosis (ALS)—A central nervous system disease of unknown etiology, almost invariably fatal.

Ankle-foot orthosis (AFO)—A brace or splint used to support the foot by stabilizing the ankle.

Antibiotic—A medication designed to kill bacteria.

Antibody— A protein made by the immune system of the body in response to a substance, usually of foreign origin, called an antigen.

Anxiety—A feeling of worry, uneasiness.

Apraxia—The inability to perform a purposeful movement even though the ability exists to perform the components of the movement.

Ataxia—The inability to properly coordinate movement. This usually refers to walking and to movement of the arms.

Autoimmune disease—A disease, such as rheumatoid arthritis or MS, that involves the immune system of the body turning against a component of the body itself.

Autonomic nervous system—The portion of the peripheral nervous system that is not under voluntary control. It governs "automatic" functions such as sweating, heart rate, sexual functions, and bowel motility

Axons—The nerves that carry impulses from a cell to another nerve cell or a muscle.

B cell—A type of white blood cell formed in the bone marrow, involved in immunologic reactions.

Babinski sign—An upward movement of the great toe on stimulating the sole of the foot that often occurs with abnormalities of the central nervous system.

Bacteria—Small organisms (germs) that can sometimes be shown to be involved in some infectious diseases and are often treated with antibiotics.

Bladder—A muscular sac that stores urine prior to urination.

Blood–brain barrier—The barrier that prevents entry of many substances into the brain from the blood vessels. A break in the blood–brain barrier may underlie the disease process in MS.

Bowel—The lowest portion of the large intestine, involved in elimination.

Brain stem—The part of the central nervous system that controls breathing and the heart; it connects the cerebrum to the spinal cord.

Bulk former—A substance that adds bulk to the stool; frequently used in the management of constipation.

Catheter, urinary—A tube inserted into the bladder for drainage of urine.

Central nervous system (CNS)—The CNS consists of the brain and spinal cord. It is where many bodily functions (such as muscle control, eyesight, breathing, memory, and so forth) are generated, processed, and signaled to the different parts of the body.

Cerebellum—The part of the brain responsible for coordinating motor movement.

Certified occupational therapy assistant (COTA)—A person trained to perform some of the duties of registered occupational therapists, usually under their supervision.

Cerebral spinal fluid—A clear fluid that surrounds and cushions the brain and spinal cord.

Clonus—Alternating contraction and relaxation of a muscle in an extremity (arm or leg), resulting in a shaking movement or spasm.

Cognition—The comprehension and use of speech, visual perceptions and construction, calculation ability, attention (information processing), memory, and executive functions such as planning, problem solving, and self-monitoring.

Colon—The lower part of the large intestine.

Computerized tomogram (CT scan)—A sophisticated X-ray that utilizes a computer to give a three-dimensional and internal view of an organ.

Condom catheter—A thin, flexible sheath connected to a tube that is worn over the penis, allowing urine to drain through the tube to a collecting system.

Constipation—The inability to relieve oneself of stool.

Continence—The ability to control urination and defecation.

Contracture—A decrease in the range of motion in a joint due to stiffness (spasticity) in the surrounding muscles.

Coping—Adjusting or adapting successfully to a challenge.

Cortisone/Corticosteroid—A hormone of the adrenal glands known to have anti-inflammatory and immune system–suppressing properties.

Credé technique—Pushing on the bladder with a closed fist through the abdominal wall to allow more complete emptying of the bladder.

Crutch, Lofstrand—A crutch with a forearm holder used for support.

Cystitis—Inflammation of the bladder that often occurs with infection.

Cystoscopy—Examination of the bladder with a special viewing device, a cystoscope.

Cytotoxic (killer) T cell—A type of white blood cell formed after mature T cells interact with antigen on a foreign cell.

Decubitus—A break in the skin resulting from pressure on an area for a prolonged period; a pressure sore.

Demyelination—The abnormal process of myelin destruction that results in disruption of the normal pattern of nerve conduction.

Depression—Altered mood characterized by feelings of gloom.

Dexamethasone (Decadron)—A high-potency cortisone used to decrease swelling (inflammation) in the nervous system.

Diplopia—Double vision.

Dizziness—The sensation of light-headedness.

Dysarthria—Slurring of speech.

Dysesthesia—Pain of a burning nature along a nerve.

Dysmetria—The inability to control the range of a voluntary muscle movement causing over/under shoot and decreased coordination.

Dysphagia—Difficulty with swallowing.

Dysphonia—Disorders of voice quality caused by spasticity, weakness, and incoordination of muscles in the mouth and throat.

Dyssynergic bladder—A type of bladder in which the urethral sphincter and the bladder wall operate in an uncoordinated fashion.

Dystrophy, muscular—A familial disease of wasting and weakness of muscles.

Dysuria—Painful urination.

Edema—Local or generalized condition in which body tissues contain an excessive amount of fluid; swelling.

Ejaculation—The ejection of semen from the penis.

Electrophoresis—The movement of charged particles through a medium that has an electrical potential associated with it.

Emotional lability—An inability to control emotions.

Encephalomyelitis—An inflammation of the brain and spinal cord.

Endemic—Referring to a disease that occurs continuously in a particular population.

Energy conservation—The careful control of energy to prevent fatigue and maximize function.

Enterostomy—The surgical formation of a permanent opening through the abdominal wall, usually following removal of a portion of the intestine or urinary tract.

Epidemiology—The study of factors in the environment that influence disease.

Etiology—The study of all factors that may be involved in the development of a disease.

Euphoria—An inappropriate feeling of well-being sometimes associated with the "cerebral" form of MS.

Evoked potentials—The stimulation of an organ (e.g., eye, ear, skin) to elicit an electrical discharge in the brain; many diseases, including MS, alter the normal pattern by which a stimulus is transmitted to the brain.

Exacerbation—A sudden worsening of symptoms.

Exercise, aerobic—Performed activity designed to increase endurance and heart–lung support.

Exercise, balance—Performed activity designed to improve coordination.

Exercise, relaxation—Performed activity designed to increase relaxation.

Experimental allergic encephalomyelitis (EAE)—A disease of animals and occasionally of humans in which an immune reaction (allergic) occurs involving the nervous system (brain and spinal cord); similar to MS in many ways.

Experimental autoimmune encephalomyelitis (EAE)—A disease created in animals that is autoimmune in nature and is similar in many respects to MS.

Extensor spasm—A symptom of spasticity in which the legs straighten suddenly into a stiff, extended position. They most commonly occur in bed at night or upon arising from bed.

Fasciculation—An involuntary contraction of muscle fibers.

Fat—A substance that is broken down by digestion into fatty acid.

Fatigue—A feeling of tiredness; MS often is associated with a lassitude that is debilitating.

Flaccidity—Looseness and accompanying weakness in an affected muscle.

Flexor spasm—A spasm of legs in a knees-bent position, often occurring with minimal stimulation.

Fluency—The smoothness of speech or movement.

Foley catheter—A tube placed in the bladder to drain urine; held in place by an inflated balloon.

Foot drop—A condition of weakness in the muscles of the foot and ankle that interferes with a person's ability to flex the ankle and walk normally. The toes touch the ground before the heel does, which causes the person to trip or lose balance.

Gait—Walking pattern, often disrupted in MS.

Gastrocnemius—Muscle of the lower leg, used for normal movement of the foot.

Genetic—Pertaining to heredity.

Gluteus maximus—Muscle of the buttock.

Hamstring—Three muscles on the posterior aspect of the thigh that flex, adduct (pull in), and extend the thigh.

Helper T cell—A type of white blood cell that enhances the production of antibody-forming cells from B lymphocytes.

Hemiplegia—A weakness of an arm and leg on the same side of the body.

Hereditary disease—A disease transmitted from one generation to another.

Hesitancy—The inability to void on command; the urge to urinate without the process occurring on command.

HLA typing—The ability to type tissues in a manner analogous to blood typing.

Hot bath test—A test occasionally used to induce MS symptoms by placing a person in a tub of hot water.

Hyperbaric oxygen—Oxygen under greater than normal atmospheric pressure.

Immune defect—The general term describing a variety of malfunctions of the immune system, in which it either does not respond to a foreign substance by destroying or neutralizing it, or in which the immune system erroneously destroys normal structures of the body. Multiple sclerosis may be the result of such a defect, with myelin the specific substance attacked.

Immune response—The reaction of the body to substances that are foreign or are interpreted as being foreign.

Immune system—Consists of a number of different organs in the human body (lymph nodes, bone marrow, thymus, and so forth) that produce certain types of white blood cells and antibodies that have the ability to destroy or neutralize various germs, substances, poisons, and other harmful substances.

Immunosuppressant drug—A medication used to decrease the level of function of the immune system.

Impotence—The inability of a male to complete the sexual act.

Incidence—The number of newly occurring cases per unit of time and unit of population.

Incontinence—The inability to control the bladder or bowels.

Incoordination—The inability to produce a harmonious, rhythmic muscular action that is not the result of weakness.

Interferon—A group of immune system proteins, produced and released by cells infected by a virus, which inhibit vital multiplication and modify the body's immune responses.

Internuclear ophthalmoplegia (INO)—An abnormality of eye movement caused by demyelination between the nerve cells that control the eye muscles; this finding is common in MS.

Irrigation of the bladder—Washing out of the bladder with fluid.

Joint—The place where two bones are joined.

Kinesiology—The study of muscles and muscular movement.

Klenzak brace—A brace made with metal supports connected to a shoe to prevent foot drop.

Labia major—The two folds lying on either side of the vaginal opening.

Labia minor—The two folds inside the opening of the vagina.

Lassitude—A specific type of fatigue occurring in MS; characterized by a feeling of overwhelming tiredness.

Laxative—A food or chemical substance that acts to treat constipation.

Lesion—A physical abnormality in the nervous system.

Lhermitte's sign—The feeling of an electrical sensation down the spine when the head is bent to the chest, often due to demyelination in the neck region of the spinal cord.

Linoleic acid—A component of myelin.

Lumbar puncture—A spinal tap, involving the insertion of a needle into the spinal canal in order to obtain spinal fluid and/or inject substances into the spinal canal.

Lyme disease—A recurrent inflammatory disorder characterized by distinctive skin rash, arthritis, and involvement of the heart and nervous system; caused by a spirochete, *Ixodes damminv*; it is tick-borne.

Lymph—The proteinaceous fluid that circulates through the body in distinct channels.

Lymphocyte—A white blood cell that is a part of the immune system; it fights foreign substances, e.g., bacteria, viruses, and so forth, and is also a prominent cell in autoimmune reactions (reactions against oneself); varieties of lymphocytes include B cells and T cells.

Lysosome—A substance in the cell that is responsible for some enzyme reactions that break down proteins.

Macrophage—A cell in the body that helps in cleansing the body of foreign substances.

Magnetic resonance imaging (MRI)—A diagnostic procedure that produces visual images of different body parts without the use of X-rays. An important diagnostic tool in MS that makes it possible to visualize and count lesions in the white matter of the brain and spinal cord.

Metabolism—Energy changes that occur within the cells of the body.

Monoclonal antibody—A specific antibody formed against a single substance by the immune system.

Monoplegia—Weakness in a single arm or leg.

Motor—Usually referring to the ability to carry out activities that require the use of bodily muscles.

Multiple sclerosis—A disorder of the CNS usually characterized by worsenings (exacerbations) and improvements (remissions) of symptoms. Multiple scars gradually form in the CNS. Most frequently encountered symptoms are loss of strength, difficulties with balance and bladder control, numbness and tingling, and blurred or double vision.

Myelin—A substance consisting of fat and protein, which acts as an insulator around most of the nerve fibers in the human body. It is found in the central and peripheral nervous systems.

Myelination/myelinization—The process of acquiring a myelin sheath.

Myelinoclasis—The destruction of the components of myelin.

Myelinolysis—The destruction of myelin sheaths.

Myelitis—Inflammation of the spinal cord.

Myelography—An examination of the spinal cord performed by the introduction of a dye into the spinal canal followed by X-rays.

Myelopathy—Any pathologic condition of the spinal cord.

Myokymia—A twitching of muscles, usually of the face, caused by increased irritability in MS.

Natural killer cells—Cells in the immune system that may play a role in MS.

Nerve—A bundle of nerve fibers (axons). The fibers are either afferent (leading toward the brain and serving in the perception of sensory stimuli of the skin, joints, muscles, and inner organs) or efferent (leading away from the brain and mediating contractions of muscles or organs).

Neuralgia—A sharp pain along the course of a nerve.

Neurogenic bladder—A condition in which urinary bladder control is disturbed, which may manifest itself by frequent urgencies for urination, a loss of sensation for urge, an inability to empty the bladder even though the urge may be present, or a complete loss of control of the urinary bladder, which then empties itself irregularly.

Neurologist—A physician who specializes in the diagnosis and treatment of diseases of the nervous system.

Neuropathy—A degeneration of the nerves to the arms, legs, or internal organs.

Nocturia—The necessity to urinate at night.

Numbness—The loss of sensation in an area of the body.

Nutrition—The body's use of food, including ingestion, digestion, and absorption.

Olfactory—The sensation involved with smell.

Oligoclonal bands—A diagnostic sign indicating abnormal levels of certain antibodies in the cerebrospinal fluid; seen in approximately 90 percent of people with MS, but not specific to MS.

Oligodendrocyte—The cell type in the central nervous system responsible for making and supporting myelin.

Optic atrophy—A wasting of the optic disc that results from partial or complete degeneration of optic nerve fibers and is associated with a loss of visual acuity.

Optic neuritis—An inflammation of the nerve that connects the eye with the brain, which manifests itself mainly as blurring or loss of vision and occasionally pain.

Orgasm—The height of excitement at the time of sexual intercourse.

Orthotist—One skilled in making mechanical appliances for preservation of function.

Paraplegia—A weakness of both legs.

Paresthesia—A sensation of tingling or "pins and needles" in different portions of the body.

Parasympathetic nervous system—The part of the autonomic nervous system that is partially responsible for automatic functions, e.g., heart, blood pressure, bladder/bowel, sexual; centered in the head and lower spinal region.

Paroxysmal spasm—A sustained contraction of a limb that is uncontrolled and occurs intermittently.

Passive stretching—The movement of a person's muscles to a stretched position by someone other than that person.

Patterning—The guiding of movements over and over to allow the brain to develop repeated functions; underlies many of the physical therapies used in MS management.

Peripheral nervous system—Numerous nerves in the body that serve the function of carrying the stimuli and information into the brain and spinal cord and, from there, back into the different parts of the body.

Physiatrist—A physician who specializes in physical medicine and rehabilitation; may be involved in the management of MS.

Placebo—An inactive substance given to group of patients in a drug study to compare with the active substance; any inactive substance given instead of an active one.

Plaque—An area of inflamed or demyelinated CNS tissue.

Plasmapheresis—The removal of plasma (the fluid of blood), with replacement by an appropriate fluid; removes impurities in the plasma.

Position sense—The ability to feel slight movements of fingers or toes.

Pressure sore—*See* Decubitus; Ulcer.

Prevalence—The algebraic product of incidence and duration (how many cases per unit of population at any one time).

Protein—A class of chemicals naturally occurring in plants and animals composed of nitrogen and amino acids.

Pyuria—Pus in the urine due to infection.

Quadriceps—Muscle of the upper leg involved in straightening of the leg.

Quadriplegia—Weakness of all four extremities (arms and legs).

Range of motion—The movement of a muscle about a joint.

Ranvier's nodes—Constrictions in the myelin sheath that allow for extremely rapid electrical transmission.

Rectum—The lowest part of the bowel, the part that follows the colon, which pushes the stool out during elimination.

Reflex—An immediate response of a certain part of the human body to a brief stimulus, which usually does not require processing of the stimulus through the conscious mind. An example is the jerking of the leg upon striking it or withdrawal from fire before conscious awareness.

Relaxation technique—A technique designed to calm, including biofeedback, meditation, or yoga.

Remission—A lessening in the severity of symptoms or their temporary disappearance during the course of the illness.

Retrobulbar neuritis—Swelling or irritation of the optic nerve behind the eye secondary to inflammation.

Romberg's sign—An inability to maintain the body balance with the eyes shut and the feet close together.

Schwann cell—The cell that makes myelin in the peripheral nervous system.

Scotoma—A blind spot in the field of vision.

Semen—The thick secretion from the urethra (penis) emitted at the climax of sexual excitement.

Sensory—Pertaining to the ability to feel, sense, taste, smell, see, and hear.

Sexuality—Related to the total sexual life of a person—whether including the sexual organs themselves or not.

Sign, clinical—A physical abnormality found on examination.

Spasticity—The loss of normal elasticity of leg and/or arm muscles resulting from a disease process in the CNS. It is often manifested by extreme stiffness of the muscles, which results in difficulties with active and passive movements of the extremities.

Sphincter—A circular band of muscle fibers that tightens or closes a natural opening of the body, such as the external anal sphincter, which closes the anus, and the internal and external urinary sphincters, which close the urinary canal.

Spinal cord—The part of the CNS that connects the brain and its related structures to the peripheral nervous system.

Spinal tap—*See* Lumbar puncture.

Steroids—Chemicals that either mimic or are from various endocrine organs of the body (usually the adrenal gland); they are potent anti-inflammatory (antiswelling) and immune-suppressing agents and often used in the management of MS.

Suppressor T cells—A type of lymphocyte that suppresses the production of antibody-forming cells from B lymphocytes.

Suprapubic catheter—A tube placed in the bladder through the skin just above the pelvic bone (pubic bone).

Sympathetic nervous system—That part of the autonomic (automatic) nervous system partially responsible for many automatic functions, such as sweating, heart beating, sexual activity, bowel/bladder function; centered in the chest and low back region.

Symptom—The subjective description of a problem as perceived by the individual.

T cell—A type of white blood cell formed in the thymus, tonsils, and other organs involved in the immunologic reaction; believed to be substantially involved in the MS process.

Tactile—Refers to the sensation involved with touch.

Therapeutic recreation specialist—A person trained to develop programs aimed at group or individual leisure activities (usually a bachelor's or master's training).

Tonic spasm—*See* Paroxysmal spasm.

Transcutaneous nerve stimulation (TNS)—The placing of an electrical stimulation along an area to stimulate the nerve in the same region—used for pain control.

Transverse myelitis—An acute attack of inflammatory demyelination in which the spinal cord loses its ability to transmit nerve impulses up and down. Paralysis and numbness are experienced in the legs and trunk below the level of the inflammation.

Tremors—Various involuntary movements involving arms, legs, or head, occurring in numerous illnesses and conditions and greatly varying in type and severity.

Trigeminal neuralgia—Severe pain in the face due to irritation of a nerve from the brain stem.

Triplegia—Weakness of three of four extremities (arms and legs)

Ulcer—An open sore (decubitus) in the skin or other membrane such as stomach or intestine.

Urethra—The canal for discharge of urine from the bladder.

Urethral sphincter—The valve controlling the flow of urine into the urethra.

Urine culture—The growing of bacteria (germs) from a specimen of urine to determine the presence and cause of an infection.

Urinary tract—The pathway involved in urination; it includes the kidneys, ureter, bladder, and urethra.

Vertigo—Dizziness or a spinning sensation.

Vestibular stimulation—The stimulation of the balance part of the ear by exercise.

Virus—A small organism (germ) with distinctive features consisting of either DNA or RNA, which is unaffected by most antibiotics and sometimes can be shown to be involved in some diseases.

Vision—The ability to see.

Vitamin—A substance essential for growth, development, and normal body processes.

Voiding—The elimination of urine or stool.

Vulva—The general term for the external female sexual organs.

Walker—A mobile device used to assist a person in walking.

Weakness—A decrease in physical strength.

Weighting—The use of weights placed on an extremity to decrease movement.

White matter—The part of the brain that contains myelinated nerve fibers and appears white, in contrast to the cortex of the brain, which contains nerve cell bodies and appears gray.

Appendix

B

EXERCISES FOR SPASTICITY

RANGE OF MOTION—LOWER EXTREMITY

CAUTION—When doing passive exercises, do them slowly and apply pressure steadily, especially if extreme tightness is present.

1. Ankle Dorsiflexion (Calf Stretch)

Bending ankle up: Back lying.

Grab the heel, placing the ball of the foot against your forearm, and bend the ankle up. (Push the toes toward the knee.)

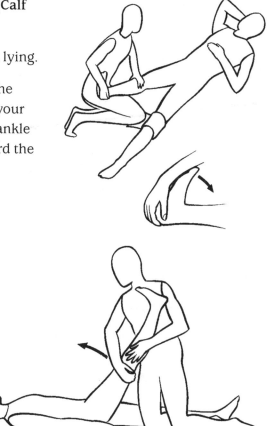

2. Hamstring Stretch

Hip flexion with straight knee: Back lying.

3. Hip Flexion

Knee to chest: Buttock stretch. Back lying.

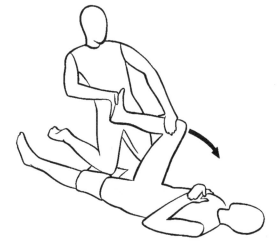

4. Internal–External Rotation

Rolling leg in and out: Back lying.

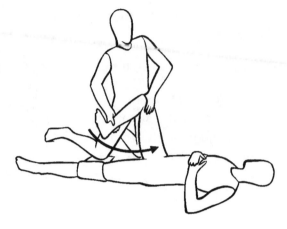

5. Abduction–Adduction

Out to side: Back lying.

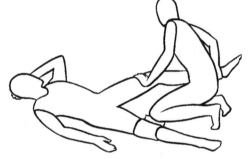

6. Knee Flexing

Front, thigh stretch: Face lying.

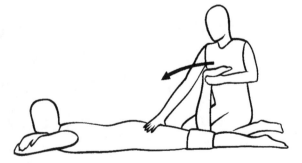

7. Hip Extension

Leg backward at hip:
Face lying.

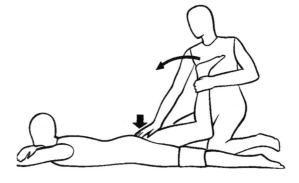

8. Trunk Flexion

Back stretch: Bring
both knees up to chest.
Back lying.

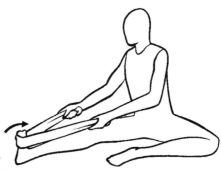

INDEPENDENT STRETCHING PROGRAM

1. Heel cord Stretch

Sit on a mat, the floor, or the
bed with your legs stretched
out in front of you. (If this is
difficult, sit with your back
against the wall.) Take a towel
and sling it around your foot,
across the ball of the foot, and
pull the forefoot up toward you.
You should feel a stretch in your
calves and up behind the knees.
Hold for 60 seconds.

2. Hamstring Stretch

Sitting as in the first exercise, lean forward, place your hands on your calves, and slide them down toward your toes, keep your knees straight. You should feel a stretch under your thighs. Try to keep your back relatively straight. Hold for 60 seconds.

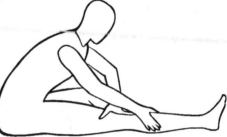

3. Butterfly Sit

Sit on the bed, floor, or mat with your knees and hips bent and the soles of your feet touching. Clasp your ankles with your hands so that your elbows rest on the inside of your knees. Push the knees apart with your elbows as you lean forward. Hold for 60 seconds.

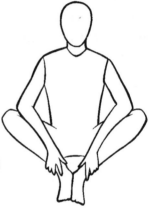

4. Wall Stretch

Lie on your back at the base of a wall—perpendicular to it (either on the floor or on a bed if it is against the wall). Your buttocks should be all the way up against the wall and your legs stretched out and up against the wall. Let the legs slowly separate and slide out to the side as far as possible. Hold for 60 seconds.

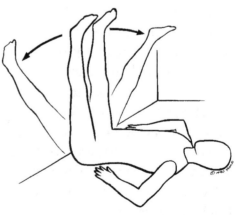

5. Kneel Standing

Get your knees on a mat or the floor. Then lower your buttocks down to the right heel and come back up. Then down to the left heel and back up again. Repeat five to seven times—progress as tolerated.

BALANCE AND COORDINATION

1. Kneeling

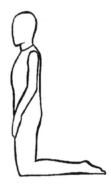

2. Sitting

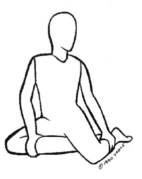

3. Four-Point Kneeling

Note equal distribution of weight over the four points of contact.

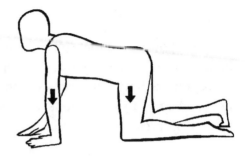

4. Stand Kneeling

This position develops increased balance by establishing pelvic and hip control.

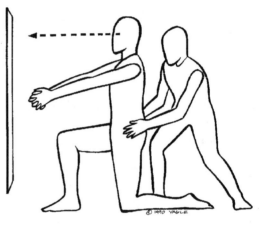

5. Turning to Look Behind

This exercise challenges the balance system.

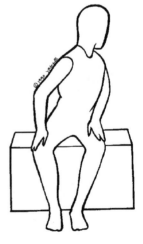

6. **Taking Weight through Affected Arm**

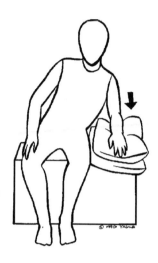

Strengthening Exercises

1. **Knee Extension**

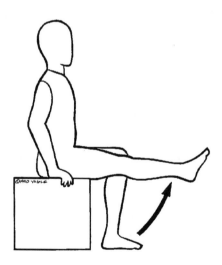

2. Quad Set

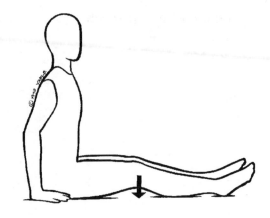

3. Terminal Knee Extension

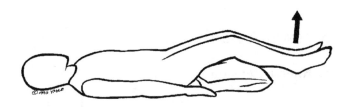

4. Elbow Flexion with Theraband

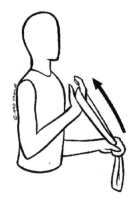

5. Elbow Extension with
   Theraband

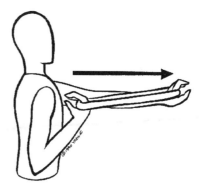

6. Shoulder Flexion–Extension with
   Theraband

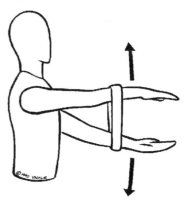

7. External Rotation with
   Theraband

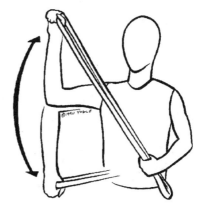

8. **Shoulder Abduction with Theraband**

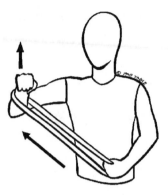

9. **Shoulder Adduction with Theraband**

10. **Exercises for Strengthening Fingers with Use of Putty.**

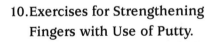

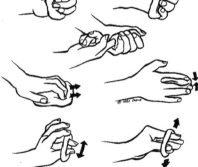

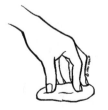

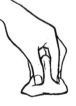

Appendix
C

TRANSFERS AND MOBILITY

WHEELCHAIR TO BED WITH SLIDING BOARD
General Tips

- Move wheelchair next to bed as close as possible.

- Remove armrest closest to bed.

- Lock wheels

- Be sure board has handles or loops on end for ease in moving.

1. Place sliding board under buttocks closest to bed at angle from front of chair seat to bed.

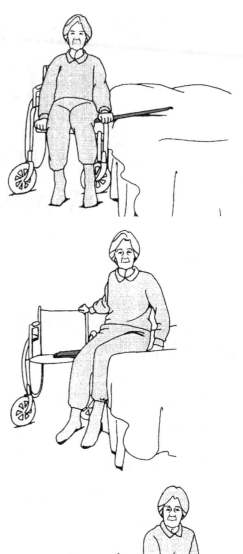

2. Push up on armrest or back of chair and slide over to bed. Establish sitting balance.

3. Bring legs up onto bed.

4. Final position.

Lean away from board and move board to safe location.

Reverse this procedure to return to wheelchair.

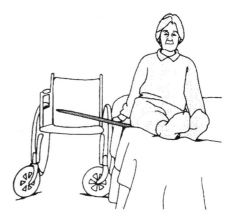

TRANSFER WHEELCHAIR TO BED (ASSISTED AS NEEDED)

1. Remove feet from footrests, move footrests out of way, lock brakes. Be sure feet are flat on ground and uninvolved foot is slightly forward. (If both legs are weak, place stronger leg slightly forward.)

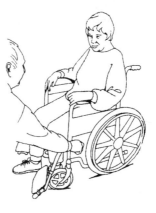

2. Lean trunk forward and push on armrest to come to standing position. (Assist if necessary.)

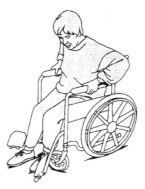

3. Balance in standing
   position for a few seconds.

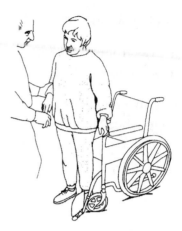

4. Pivot the feet until the
   backs of the legs are
   against the bed.

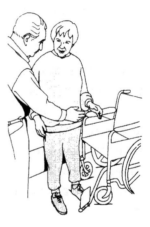

5. Slowly lower body onto
   bed while bending knees.
   If possible, use arms to
   assist with lowering.

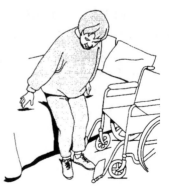

6. Left each leg onto the bed.

(Assist if necessary.)

Reverse this procedure to
return to wheelchair.

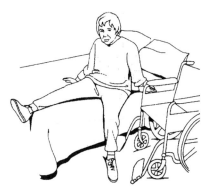

Transfer Wheelchair to Car (Assisted)

General Tips

- Open the car door.
- Position wheelchair as close as possible (leave enough room for helper and person to stand and pivot). See picture #1.
- Remove feet from footrests, move footrests out of way, lock the brakes.
- Put feet flat on the ground. Place the uninvolved foot slightly behind the involved foot.
- If both legs are weak, put the stronger leg slightly forward.
- Be sure to explain the procedure to the person you are helping before you begin.

1. Starting position.

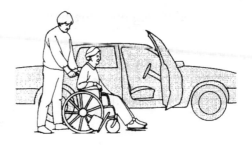

2. Help person to standing
   position. Let person
   balance a few seconds.

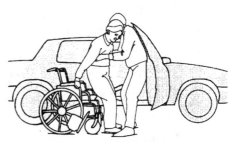

3. Help person to pivot so
   the backs of legs are
   against the seat.

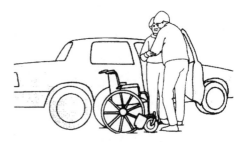

4. **Slowly lower person to sitting position.**

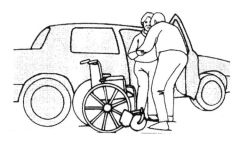

5. **Lift each leg into the car.**

Reverse the procedure to return the person to the wheelchair.

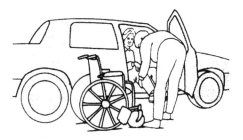

Transfer Wheelchair to Car (Unassisted)

General Tips

- Open the car door.
- Angle wheelchair as close as possible (leave enough room for person to stand and pivot). See picture #1.
- Remove feet from footrests, move footrests out of way, lock the brakes.
- Put feet flat on the ground. Place the uninvolved foot slightly behind the involved foot.
- If both legs are weak, put the stronger leg slightly forward.
- Loops or other devices may be attached to car to assist movement.

1. Starting position.

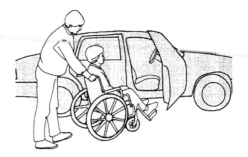

2. Lean forward, push down on armrests and come to a standing position. Balance, standing, for a few seconds.

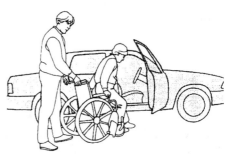

3. Pivot on feet until the backs of the legs are against the seat.

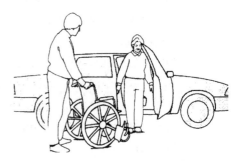

4. Slowly lower body into seat. Use the arms on the seat if possible.

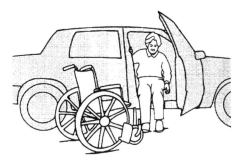

5. Lift each leg into the car.

Reverse the procedure to return to the wheelchair.

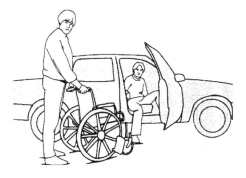

BED MOBILITY BASICS

How to Get Up from a Lying Position (Assisted as Necessary)

1. Bend knees until feet are flat.

Helper assist as needed.

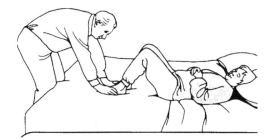

2. Lift arm closest to the side of the bed over head.

Assist as needed.

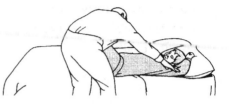

3. Roll onto side.

Assist as needed. Remind person to tighten buttocks and squeeze abdomen while rolling over.

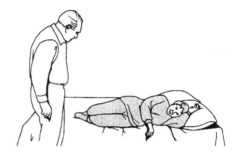

4. Push with arms and let legs hang over side of the bed until feet are flat on floor. Tighten buttocks and squeeze abdomen.

The helper can bring legs down and place hand under the shoulder to help person lift up from the trunk.

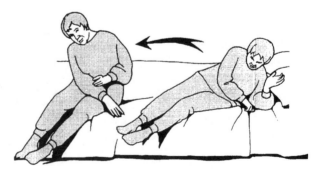

5. Sit and balance yourself.
   Relax buttocks and
   abdomen.

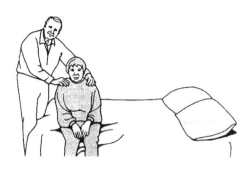

Helper should place both
hands on shoulders until the
person is stable. If unstable,
do not let go.

How to Move from Sitting to Lying
(For Person with Pain and Weakness)

1. Tighten buttocks and
   squeeze abdomen
   throughout.

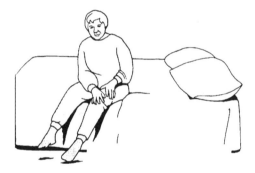

2. Lean weight onto the
   elbow of the side on
   which you will lie.

Helper assist as needed.

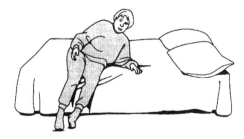

3. Bring legs onto bed while tightening buttocks and squeezing abdomen. Slide into side lying position with knees bent.

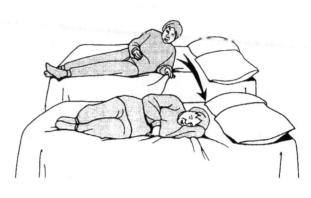

Helper assist as needed.

4. Roll onto back.

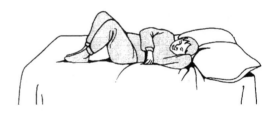

Helper assist as needed. Remind person to squeeze buttocks and tighten abdomen when beginning to roll.

5. Tighten buttocks and abdomen. Let legs slide into flattened position.

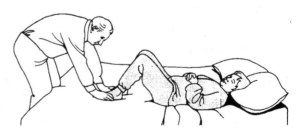

Helper may need to assist person to flatten legs.

GETTING UP FROM THE FLOOR

1. Near a piece of furniture get onto your hands and knees.

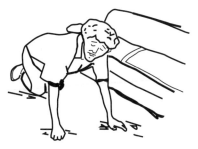

2. Facing the furniture, push up onto your knees.

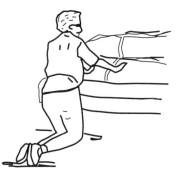

3. Assist with one hand to bring your strongest leg up.

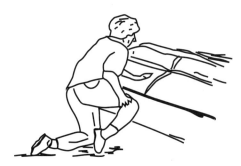

4. Place your foot flat on
   the floor.

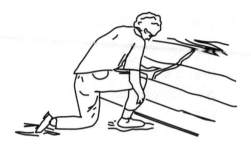

5. Lean forward and using
   your arms and legs push
   up to half-stand.

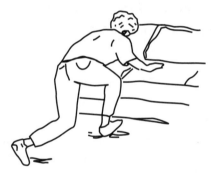

6. Turn and sit on the
   furniture.

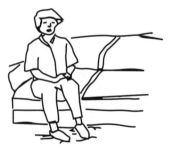

Hoyer Transfer

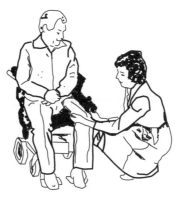

To place sling under patient, stand in front of patient, lean patient forward on knees, place sling behind patient, and bring leg flaps alongside patient's thighs. Tuck back edge of commode opening under patient's buttocks. Lean patient back. Grasp snap hook bar in one hand and, reaching under patient's leg, grasp D ring in other and pull until front edge of sling is just behind knees. Repeat on other side. Attach snap hook on each side of D ring on other side. (Can also criss-cross flaps under one leg and over the other, or support each leg independently by connecting snap hook and D ring on the same side together.)

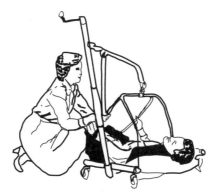

To lift patient from the floor, place sling under patient using "Z" fold as for bed pickup. Bring lifter behind patient and support patient's head and neck on pillow placed over litter base. Lower cradle so that chains reach hooks of sling. Raise patient's knees and attach sling. Lift patient.

To lower patient to floor, reverse the procedure.

$\mathcal{A}\ p\ p\ e\ n\ d\ i\ x$
D

RESOURCES

ADDITIONAL READING

Bowling AC (2007). *Complementary and Alternative Medicine and Multiple Sclerosis, Second Edition.* New York: Demos.

Coyle PK, Halper J (2007). *Living with Progressive Multiple Sclerosis, Second Edition.* New York: Demos.

Fishman LM, Small E (2007). *Yoga and Multiple Sclerosis: A Journey to Health and Healing.* New York: Demos.

Holland NJ, Reingold SC, Murray TJ (2012). *Multiple Sclerosis: A Guide for the Newly Diagnosed, Fourth Edition.* New York: Demos.

Holland N, Halper J (2005). *Multiple Sclerosis: A Self-Care Guide to Wellness, Second Edition.* New York: Demos.

Kalb RC (2011). *Multiple Sclerosis: The Questions You Have—The Answers You Need, Fifth Edition.* New York: Demos.

Kalb RC (2005). *Multiple Sclerosis: A Guide for Families, Third Edition.* New York: Demos.

Kalb RC, Geisser B, Holland NJ (2012). *MS for Dummies* (2nd Edition). Hoboken, NJ: Wiley.

Kraft GH, Catanzaro M (2000). *Living with Multiple Sclerosis: A Wellness Approach, Second Edition.* New York: Demos.

Lechtenberg R (1995). *Multiple Sclerosis Fact Book.* Philadelphia: Davis.

LeMaistre J (1994). *Beyond Rage: Mastering Unavoidable Health Changes.* Dillon, CO: Alpine Guild.

Northrop D, Cooper S (2007). *Health Insurance Resources: Options for People with a Chronic Illness or Disability, Second Edition.* New York: Demos.

Peterman Schwarz S (2006). *Multiple Sclerosis: 300 Tips for Making Life Easier, Second Edition.* New York: Demos.

Polman CH, Thompson AJ, Murray TJ, McDonald WI (2006). *Multiple Sclerosis: The Guide to Treatment and Management, Sixth Edition.* New York: Demos.

Vazquez TC, DeThomas PF (2001). *Esclerosis Múltiple: Guia para el Recién Diagnosticado.* New York: Demos.

ELECTRONIC INFORMATION SOURCES

Some of the best sources of information about MS available on the Internet are:

- National Multiple Sclerosis Society: www.nmss.org
- Multiple Sclerosis Association of America (MSAA): www.mymsaa.org
- Multiple Sclerosis Society of Canada: www.mssoc.ca
- Multiple Sclerosis Society of Canada/Société canadienne: www.mssociety.ca
- Multiple Sclerosis International Federation: www.msif.org
- Consortium of Multiple Sclerosis Centers: www.mscare.org
- Can Do MS: www.mscando.org
- Eastern Paralyzed Veterans Association: www.epva.org
- Paralyzed Veterans of America: www.pva.org
- ABLEDATA: www.abledata.com.

INDEX

Index

oligodendrocytes (oligos), 6
onabotulinumtoxin A (Botox), 86
ondansetron (Zofran), 60, 61
optic nerve, 108
optic neuritis, 108–109
oral motor exercises, 102–104
organizations, 20
orthopedic exercises, 114
orthoses, 47, 67
osteoporosis, 156
overweight, 136
oxcarbazepine (Trileptal), 65

paceboards, 63, 104
pain, 110–114
pain clinics, 112
parasympathetic nervous system, 5, 6
Parkinson's disease, 49, 63
paroxetine (Paxil), 37
paroxysmal (tonic) spasms, 51
paroxysmal symptoms, 64–65
passive stretching, 46
patience, 20
patient empowerment, 26–27
patterning, 59
pemoline (Cylert), 37
penile vacuum devices, 147–148
penis, 144
percutaneous rhizotomy, 110–111
Peri-Colace, 100
peripheral nervous system (PNS), 4, 5
personalities, 19
personality changes, 152
phenol, 51
phenothiazine tranquilizers, 61
phenytoin (Dilantin), 64, 110
physiatrists, 15
physical therapy, for vertigo, 116
physician
    choosing your, 14–17
    disease management philosophy
        of, 25
    expectations about, 16
physician–patient relationship, 17–18
physician's assistants, 15
physiologic tremors, 61
plaques, 6
plasma exchange, 26, 31
polypeptides, 22
pools, 46
postural muscles, 44
potassium channel blockers, 36

power chairs, 66
pramipexole dihydrochloride
    (Mirapex), 48, 49
prednisone, 30
pregabalin (Lyrica), 50, 65, 111
pregnancy, 13
pressure sores, 74–76
primary progressive MS, 8
primary symptoms, 33–34
primidone (Mysoline), 60, 61
progressive multifocal
    leukoencephalopathy (PML), 24,
    29–30
progressive muscle relaxation, 47
progressive-relapsing MS, 8
progressive resistive exercises, 54–55
propranolol (Inderal), 60
prostaglandin, 147
proteins, 128
pumps, 52

quad set, 186

raising children, 155
range of motion exercise, 178–181
range of movement, 46
rectal stimulants, 100–101
rectum, 95
rehabilitation, 26
relapses, 31
relapsing-remitting MS, 8
relaxation exercises, 140
relaxation techniques, 47, 153–155
remission, 7
resting tremors, 61
restless legs, 35, 49
retrobulbar neuritis, 108–109
rheumatoid arthritis, 11
ropinirole (Requip), 48, 49
rubella, 12
rubeola, 12

Sativex, 50
saturated fats, 128
sclerotic (scarred) areas, 3
scooters, 70–73
secondary progressive MS, 8
secondary symptoms, 34
self-catheterization, 87–88, 90
self-esteem, 150, 151
sertraline (Zoloft), 37
sexual functioning, 142–143

Index

ABOUT THE AUTHOR

Randall (Randy) T. Schapiro, MD was born and raised in Minnesota. After graduating from Occidental College (Los Angeles, CA) in Biology, he graduated from the University of Minnesota Medical School. He trained in internal medicine at the Wadsworth VA Medical Center (UCLA) in Los Angeles and then in neurology under A. B. Baker, MD at the University of Minnesota. Following a short stint as a faculty member and director of the MS Clinic at the University of Minnesota he founded the first private practice comprehensive MS Center in 1977, The Fairview MS Center, which was renamed, The Schapiro Center for Multiple Sclerosis at the Minneapolis Clinic of Neurology in 2004.

He was the first elected president of the Consortium of MS Centers, an organization which he helped found. He has participated in the development of the Heuga Center (now called Can Do MS), a wellness center for MS based in Colorado and was given their "Can Do" award. He has been elected to the National MS Society Hall of Fame and has served on numerous advisory committees for them including the Medical Advisory Board. He recently was presented the prestigious Starfish Award by the National MS Society and the Lifetime Achievement Award by the Consortium of MS Centers. He also serves on the International MS Society's Medical Advisory Board. He has served five years on the National Board of the National MS Society as well as 34 years on the Minnesota board of the NMSS. He is currently on the Colorado Board.

He has lectured and written extensively on all topics associated with MS Management nationally and internationally. He retired from private practice in 2009 to devote more time to teaching and consulting on topics related to MS, including serving as Marketing & Patient Education Programming Director for Neurodegenerative Diseases at EMD Serono, Inc. While he has participated in numerous research studies he is best known for his educating and patient management style often using humor to teach some sensitive topics.